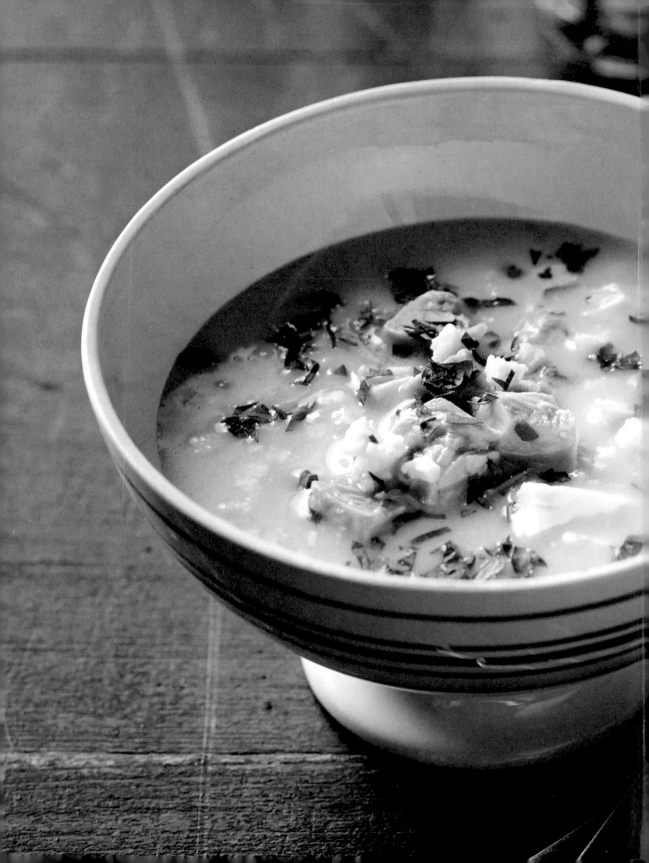

KETOFAST
COOKBOOK

ALSO BY DR. JOSEPH MERCOLA

*KetoFast**

*Superfuel**

*Fat for Fuel**

*The Fat for Fuel Ketogenic Cookbook (with Pete Evans)**

Effortless Healing

The No-Grain Diet

Sweet Deception

Dark Deception

The Great Bird Flu Hoax

Freedom at Your Fingertips

Generation XL

Healthy Recipes for Your Nutritional Type

*Available from Hay House

—

ALSO BY PETE EVANS

*The Fat for Fuel Ketogenic Cookbook (with Dr. Joseph Mercola)**

The Complete Gut Health Cookbook

The Paleo Chef

*Available from Hay House
Please visit:

Hay House USA: www.hayhouse.com®
Hay House Australia: www.hayhouse.com.au
Hay House UK: www.hayhouse.co.uk
Hay House India: www.hayhouse.co.in

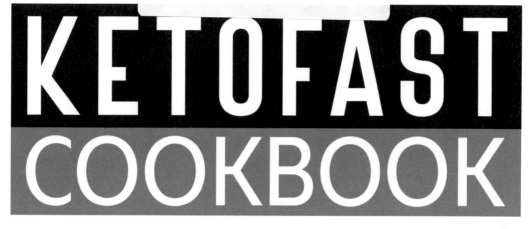

KETOFAST COOKBOOK

RECIPES FOR INTERMITTENT FASTING
AND TIMED KETOGENIC MEALS
FROM A WORLD-CLASS DOCTOR AND AN
INTERNATIONALLY RENOWNED CHEF

DR. JOSEPH MERCOLA
AND PETE EVANS

HAY HOUSE, INC.

Carlsbad, California | New York City
London | Sydney | New Delhi

Published in the United States by: Hay House, Inc.: www.hayhouse.com®
Published in Australia by: Hay House Australia Pty. Ltd.: www.hayhouse.com.au
Published in the United Kingdom by: Hay House UK, Ltd.: www.hayhouse.co.uk
Published in India by: Hay House Publishers India: www.hayhouse.co.in

Cover design: theBookDesigners
Interior design: Charles McStravick
Interior photos: William Meppem, Steve Brown, and Mark Roper (except for images used on pages 5, 6, 12, 16, 28, 32, 40, and 169 under license from Shutterstock.com)
Food stylists: Lucy Tweed and Debora Kaloper
Indexer: Jay Kreider

Library of Congress Cataloging-in-Publication Data

Names: Mercola, Joseph, author. | Evans, Pete, 1973- author.
Title: Ketofast cookbook / Dr. Joseph Mercola and Pete Evans.
Description: Carlsbad, California : Hay House, Inc., [2019] | Includes
   bibliographical references and index.
Identifiers: LCCN 2019000166| ISBN 9781401957537 (hardcover) | ISBN
   9781401957544 (e-book)
Subjects: LCSH: Fasting--Health aspects. | Cooking. | Ketogenic diet. |
   Low-carbohydrate diet--Recipes. | Lipids in human nutrition. | Health. |
   LCGFT: Cookbooks.
Classification: LCC RM226.5 .M47 2019 | DDC 641.5/6383--dc23 LC record available
at https://lccn.loc.gov/2019000166

Hardcover ISBN: 978-1-4019-5753-7
e-book ISBN: 978-1-4019-5754-4

10 9 8 7 6 5 4 3 2 1
1st edition, May 2019

To my Mom and Dad, whom I recently lost.
Thank you both for raising me.
I wouldn't be where I am today without
your love and support.

— Dr. Mercola

To all the people wanting to take health into
their own hands. Cook with love and laughter.
— Pete Evans

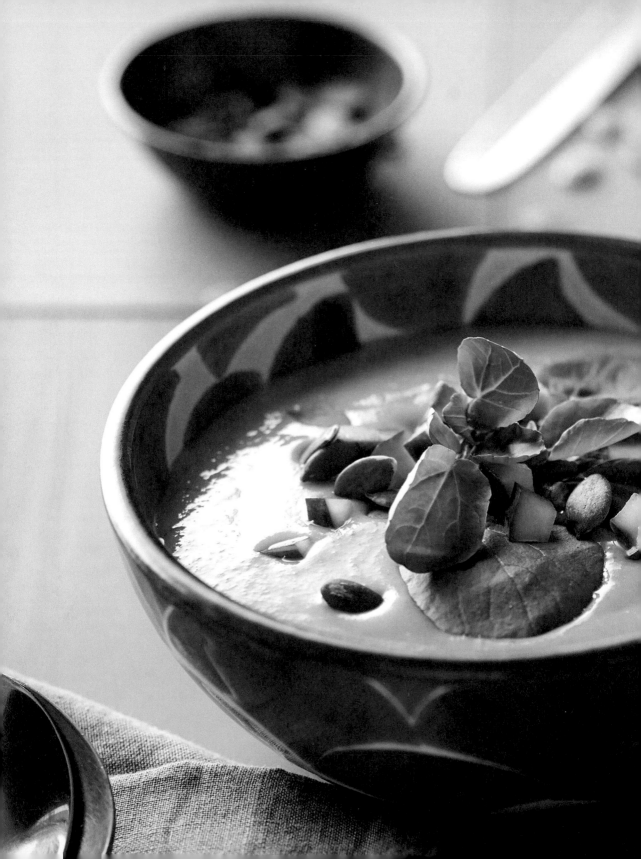

CONTENTS

||||||||||||||||||||||||||||||||||||||||||||||||||||||||||||||||||||||||||||

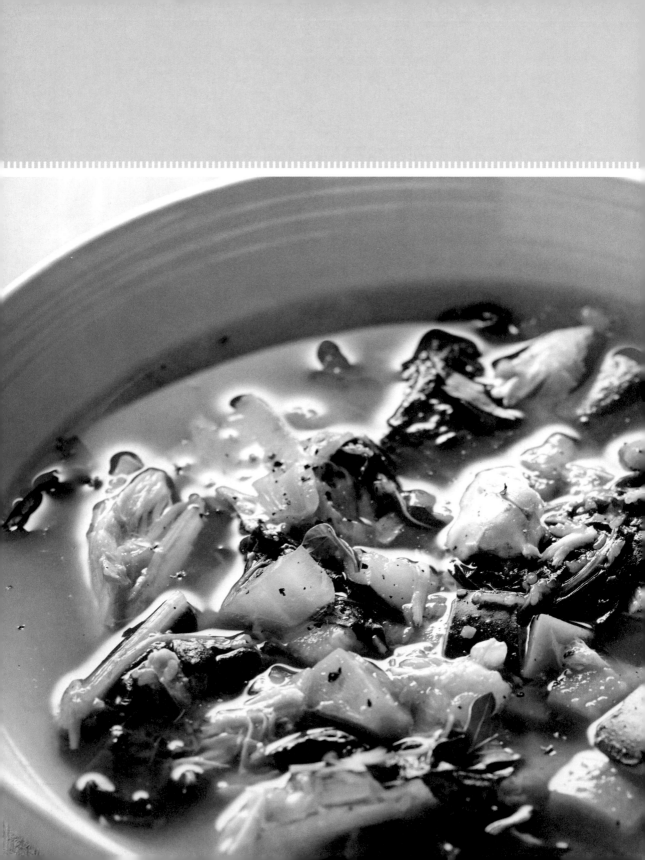

PART I

KETOFASTING

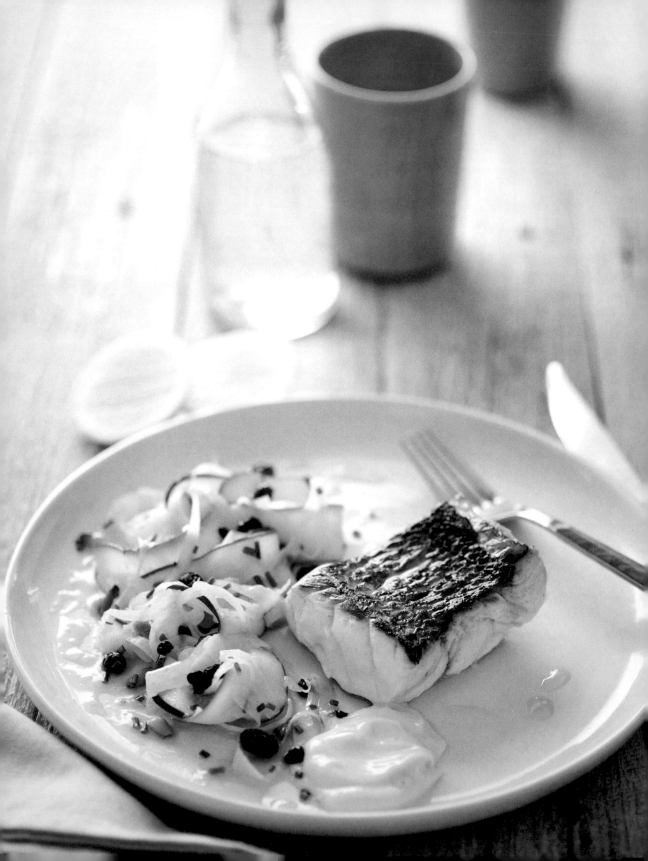

INTRODUCTION TO FASTING

I know what you might be thinking: *Why do I need a cookbook to show me what to eat when I'm fasting?* It's a perfectly valid question. After all, fasting is about not eating—so why do you need to cook anything?

Not so long ago, I also thought that "fasting" meant not eating anything. You merely stopped having food at one point, and started eating it again at another point, with nothing but water, or perhaps a cup of coffee with coconut oil, or a bowl of broth, or vegetable juice passing between your lips in the meantime. But then I began carefully studying this topic and collaborating with researchers and clinicians who have been investigating and implementing the therapeutic practice of fasting. I started to see that while true fasts—where you consume no solid food for a specific period of time—did offer some profound health benefits, they could also expose you to some perils.

This journey I've been traveling has shown me that fasting and health are, in many ways, very similar to exercise and fitness. Just as you wouldn't get up from the couch and head outside to run a marathon on your first outing, you need to work your way up to going without food—particularly if you have been eating the way most Americans do. That is to say, relying on heavily processed, carb-rich foods and eating at all hours of the day and night. These eating habits have trained your body to burn glucose as your primary fuel, which leaves you exposed to increased free radical damage, insulin resistance, and nutritional deficiencies. All of these, in turn, make it harder for you to reap the therapeutic benefits of fasting.

While fasting can and does cue your body's innate healing response, causing metabolic and cellular changes that support optimal health, it can also release chemicals and other toxins that have been safely tucked away in your fat cells. When you curtail your food intake, you enter a fasted state, which means that your body has to turn to its stores of energy for fuel, and you encourage your body to switch from burning glucose (which is derived from the carbohydrates and, to a lesser extent, the proteins you eat) to burning fat for fuel. In a fasted state, the fat that is burned comes from your fat stores. In addition to the energy that is released from the fat, the toxins that were stored in your fat cells can enter your bloodstream and wreak havoc on your body, likely contributing to many of the side effects people commonly experience when fasting, such as headaches, brain fog, and nausea.

Fat tissue has been shown to be a virtually limitless storage closet for fat-soluble toxins known by the classification *persistent organic pollutants* (POPs).[1] Once stashed away, POPs can affect the quality and quantity of overall fat tissue, making it easier to gain and harder to lose fat. POPs can also contribute to overall inflammation in your body, which has many negative effects on your metabolism and your overall health.

Multiple studies have shown that loss of fat tissue—either due to changes in your diet or from bariatric surgery—results in an increase of POPs in your blood.[2, 3] While your body does have the capability to process and eliminate these toxins once they are liberated—in fact, weight loss has been shown to reduce the total POP body burden for certain contaminants by 15 percent[4]—a sudden influx of toxins released from your fat cells can easily overwhelm your systems of detoxification, resulting in even greater damage.

What the vast majority of people need is a *gradual* approach to fasting, in which you thoughtfully change your habits—both what you eat and when—and acclimate yourself gently to the state of being able to burn fat for fuel. At the outset, you start intermittent fasting (reducing the window time during which you eat) and begin following a cyclical ketogenic diet (a high-fat, low-net-carb, moderate-protein diet, like the one I outlined extensively in my book *Fat for Fuel*). You're compressing your eating window to six to eight hours, while limiting your carbs and proteins and replacing the missing calories with high-quality fats.

Once you are metabolically flexible and able to burn fat as your primary fuel, then you can begin to add in one day a week of a partial fast—where you consume 300 to 600 calories (depending on your lean body mass) that provide the nutrients your body needs to detox effectively. Ideally you consume these calories in one single meal after your 16- to 18-hour intermittent fast ends, and then your next meal is 24 hours later. After 24 hours you have a full day of food with extra carbs and protein to supply the fuel for all the rebuilding that will be occurring in your cells as they start to regenerate after the partial fast. I call this plan Keto-Fasting, and it enables you to reap the benefits of fasting while minimizing the downsides.

To make KetoFasting as supportive of detoxification as possible, I have read hundreds of studies to get a better understanding of the nutrient-dense foods and supplements that are best for facilitating the process that carries harmful substances out of your body. And to make these foods as delicious as possible, I reached out to chef, restaurateur, and my collaborator on the *Fat for Fuel Cookbook*, Pete Evans, to create recipes that will provide the calories for your partial-fast days.

I gave Pete the nutritional parameters for the low-calorie meals that are appropriate for the days you do a partial fast, and he developed more than 40 recipes that follow those guidelines so that you have access to a variety of delicious options for the days when you are partially fasting.

For a much more complete guide to cyclical ketosis, refer to *Fat for Fuel* and the *Fat for Fuel Ketogenic Cookbook*. For a deeper dive into KetoFasting, see the companion to this cookbook, *KetoFast*. And because I am continually educating myself and refining my approach to health, be sure to sign up for my e-mail newsletter at mercola.com. When you do, you'll receive the coverage of my interviews with top researchers and practical advice for implementing their findings in your life.

It is my hope that the information on these pages you hold in your hand, as well as my other recent titles (and e-mail newsletters), will help you find your optimal level of health, and that the recipes included here will help you enjoy, and even look forward to, your fast days.

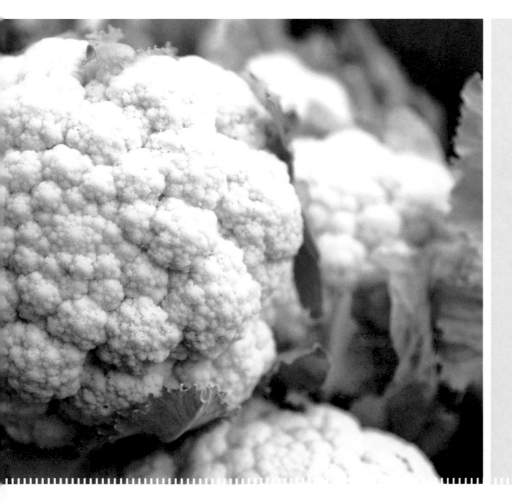

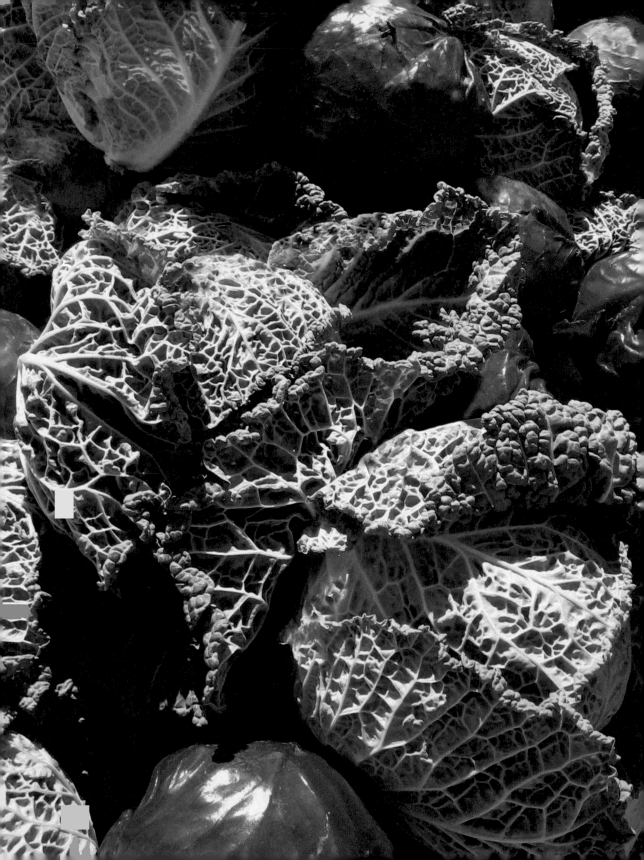

FASTING THROUGH THE AGES

I know that fasting may seem like a fad, right up there with low-fat and gluten-free, but it is not a new phenomenon or a flash in the pan. It is actually an ancient tried-and-true healing strategy that has been integral to the survival of the human race.

The truth is, up until just about 150 years ago, most of our ancestors couldn't rely on regular access to food, and a significant number of those alive today still feel this unpredictability. Humans have sometimes fasted because we don't have a choice. But humans have also known for thousands of years that periodically going without food provides a wide variety of benefits, whether health-related, mental, or even spiritual.

Major religions that observe regular fasting include:

- **Judaism.** The Talmud, a sacred Jewish text written around the 3rd century B.C.E., references several communal fasting days including Yom Kippur and Tisha B'Av, which are day-long dry fasts.

- **Christianity.** Think of Lent, the 40-day partial fast undertaken in memory of Jesus's 40-day fast.

- **Islam.** During the month-long Ramadan, Muslims abstain from food and drink from sunup to sundown.

- **Buddhism.** Some Buddhist monks, such as from the Theravada sect, eat only one meal a day.

Fasting for better health has been recommended at least since the time of ancient Greece. Plato, Plutarch, and Hippocrates—widely heralded as the father of modern medicine—all hailed the health-promoting effects of fasting. Plato wrote, "I fast for greater physical and mental efficiency." Plutarch declared, "Instead of using medicine, better fast today." And Hippocrates said about fasting, "To eat when you are sick is to feed your sickness."

Great American thinkers have praised fasting, too, including Benjamin Franklin, who said, "The best of all medicines is resting and fasting," and Mark Twain, who wrote, "A little starvation can really do more for the average sick man than can the best medicines and the best doctors."

Fasting for better health has been part of the American medical landscape since at least 1811, when Isaac Jennings, regarded as the first physician in the

United States to use therapeutic fasting in lieu of medicinal drugs, started the Natural Hygiene movement. Sylvester Graham, a Presbyterian minister, proponent of healthy living, and creator of the graham cracker, helped popularize Jennings' teachings.

In 1928, Herbert M. Shelton, D.C., N.D., founded a fasting institution and health school that provided services for more than 40 years. He also published numerous books on fasting and Natural Hygiene and developed a fasting protocol that specified consuming only water, avoiding enemas, exercise, or treatments, and observing complete rest. This is the foundation of the therapeutic fasting protocol used by Dr. Alan Goldhamer—a consultant on my book *KetoFast*—at his TrueNorth Health Center, which has overseen 16,000 people as they have undergone extended water fasting.

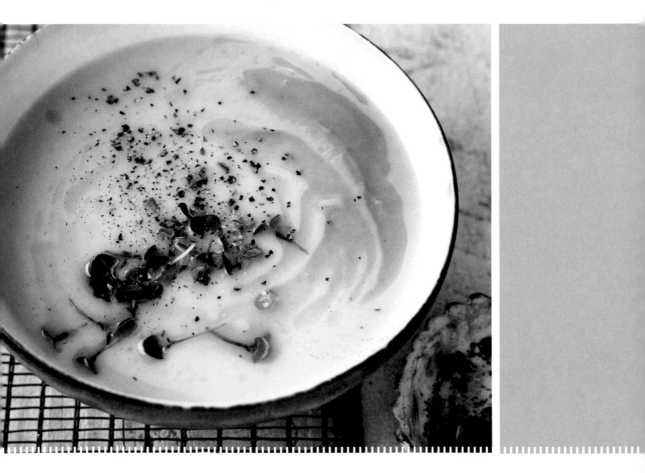

A TOUR THROUGH THE DIFFERENT TYPES OF FASTING

There are nearly as many different ways to fast as there are ways to eat. Because there are so many different approaches, and so much information is available on the Internet on the best ways to fast, I want to give an overview here so that you will be better equipped to discern the right approach for you and better able to understand why I landed on KetoFasting.

There are three basic categories of fasting:

- **Time-restricted eating (TRE),** or a type of intermittent fasting that I call Peak Fasting. It is the practice of limiting your food intake to a certain window of time each day, generally somewhere between six and eight hours. If you are new to changing your eating habits for improved health, Peak Fasting is your first step. It will help your body regain the ability to burn fat for fuel and become metabolically flexible.

  I believe that Peak Fasting is one intervention that most everyone would benefit from.

It doesn't really disrupt your normal daily experience (you may even find that you enjoy the extra time in the mornings when you don't have to worry about eating breakfast before you leave the house). And even if you don't make any other dietary changes, you can experience important health improvements.

As with all types of fasting, it's best to introduce Peak Fasting gradually. You can start by not eating anything for the three hours before you go to bed. Then, gradually, over a period of weeks or perhaps a month or two, you can delay your first meal of the day until you have reduced your window of eating down to six to eight hours—for example, eat your first meal at 11 A.M. and finish your final meal by 7 P.M. My typical eating schedule is 9 or 10 A.M. to 3 or 4 P.M.

When you eat all day long, from shortly after you wake up until just before you go to bed, you rarely, if ever, empty your glycogen stores.

It takes about 24 to 36 hours to sufficiently deplete the sugar stored in your body as glycogen, so if you don't do Peak Fasting, you will rarely, if ever, give your body the conditions it needs to start burning fat for fuel. Once you have made this metabolic switch, it will be even easier for you to go longer periods without eating.

- **Partial fasting.** In a partial fast, you greatly reduce the number of calories you eat in a day to approximately 300 to 600 (based on your lean body mass) so that you get the physiological benefits of a fast, like activating autophagy (your body's process of eliminating damaged cells by digesting them) and stem cells to help repair and regenerate your body. KetoFasting is a partial fast, and the foods that make up the few calories you're

taking in help you process any fat-soluble toxins that might be released in your body during your fasting process.

- **Water-only fasting.** This type of fasting is just as it sounds—you consume only water for the duration of the fast. This is generally done for a specific therapeutic reason, such as a serious disease or other health condition. It can be a very powerful intervention, and many people may want to consider this approach, but it is an advanced technique and I believe it should only be done either with the supervision of a health-care provider who has extensive experience in therapeutic fasting or at a dedicated fasting facility. Visit www. healthscience.org/education/ fasting/where-fast for a list of clinicians trained in this process.

One of the biggest health worries about fasting—beyond the fear of being hungry—is that your body will start consuming its own muscle tissue in an effort to get the fuel it needs to keep running.

Yet the majority of humans have enough reserves of body fat to safely undergo an extended, water-only fast for at least 40 days. In the simplest terms, the more body fat you have, the longer you will be able to fast. It is only when fat stores have been exhausted that the body turns to consuming tissues and lean muscle. But again, this happens only after fat stores are depleted, and most people can live about 40 days without food.

THE DETOXIFICATION PARADOX

As beneficial as fasting can be, there is one potential downside. When you are in a fasted state and your body begins to burn your stores of body fat for fuel, more than just energy is released, as I mentioned earlier. Toxins that have been stored in your fat tissue are liberated when the fat is burned. Those toxins then get released into your cells.

The sad truth is that we live in a toxic world and we are all exposed to potentially health-threatening toxins every day. They are in the air we breathe, the food we eat, and the water we drink—as a result of fossil fuel burning, industrial processes, chemical fertilizers and pesticides, and more.

To help you get an idea of the scope of this toxic exposure and the degree to which industry hides this information from you, I would strongly encourage you to watch the documentary *Stink* (which, as I write this, is streaming on Netflix). The documentary will provide you with an enlightening perspective on how common and dangerous these exposures are.

The good news is that your body has a brilliant protective mechanism that takes the toxins that you are exposed to and locks them away in your fat cells where they can't cause damage to your vital organs. The potentially bad news is that when you burn that fat, as fasting encourages your body to do, those toxins are freed from their protected storage spot and you are essentially exposed all over again.

Some of the harmful substances that have been shown to lurk in your fat cells include organochlorine pesticides

(OCPs), polychlorinated biphenyls (PCBs), polycyclic aromatic hydrocarbons (PAHs), and polybrominated diphenyl ethers (PBDEs). These are broadly called persistent organic pollutants (POPs).[1] Additionally, there are toxic heavy metals such as arsenic, cadmium, and lead,[2] and artificial sweeteners such as aspartame and sucralose (Splenda). In order to usher these chemicals out of your body after they have been liberated, you need to do two things:

- Support your body's ability to transform these toxins from fat-soluble into a water-soluble form so that they can be eliminated by your body.

- Encourage sweating, urination, and passing stools by doing things such as using a near-infrared sauna,

drinking plenty of high-quality liquids to improve hydration and promote urination, and ingesting substances such as fiber and the binders listed on page 45 that can absorb the toxins and sweep them out through the GI tract.

I believe it is vital to consume some well-chosen nutrients on your fast days so that your fasting has only positive effects on your health. If you are deficient in any of the nutrients that support the detoxification pathways, this process can be interrupted and the toxins can remain in your body.

This is why I suggest you follow the KetoFast protocol—to give your body the nutrients it needs to effectively break down and eliminate the harmful toxins that are stored in your fat cells.

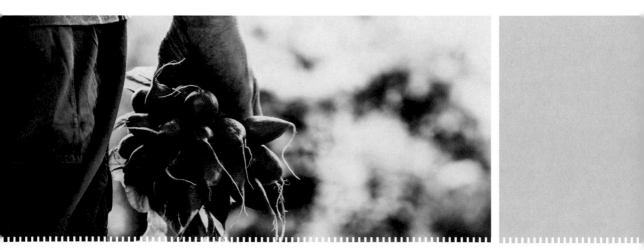

HOW TO KETOFAST

The first step I recommend in starting your KetoFast journey is to stop eating three hours before bedtime. Eating before you go to sleep tasks your body with digesting at a time when it is geared to perform functions of repair and regeneration instead. It also provides calories at a time when your energy needs are lowest, so the energy derived from that food tends to be stored as fat. But perhaps more important, the fuel backs up in your system and burns very inefficiently, resulting in an excess of potentially harmful free radicals. These free radicals then damage the DNA, cell membranes, and proteins in your cells and mitochondria, the organelles within your cells where energy is manufactured. When you give yourself a few hours to digest your food well before you go to sleep, you support your body's natural housekeeping processes. You also give your body more of a chance to deplete its glycogen stores overnight, which encourages the switch to burning fat.

Once you are used to avoiding food for at least three hours before going to sleep, your next step is to begin implementing Peak Fasting, and gradually reduce your window of eating down to six to eight hours a day. Peak Fasting will further encourage your body to manufacture and burn ketones, and enhance your rest and repair functions.

While you are going through the process of gradually expanding your Peak Fasting, you should also be eating a ketogenic diet—that is, a low-net-carb, high-fat, moderate-protein diet (as described in my book *Fat for Fuel*) that gets you into a state known as ketosis where you are burning fatty acids, known as ketones, for fuel.

Once you know you are in ketosis—because you are monitoring your ketones with either a blood or urine monitor—you can begin cycling in one or two higher-net-carb and protein days each week while also honoring a restricted six-to-eight-hour eating window. Ideally on these days you'll be doing exercise that includes some form of strength training.

This cycle of eating a ketogenic diet for five or six days a week and eating more carbs one or two days a week is known as cyclical ketosis. The ketogenic aspect of the diet is designed to improve many vital markers of your health, such as your fasting glucose and insulin levels, while adding in regular "feast" days, when you consume more carbs, helps you maintain these benefits over the long term. (The cookbook Pete Evans and I collaborated on in 2017, *Fat for Fuel Ketogenic*

Cookbook, contains nearly 100 recipes that support the guidelines of a cyclical ketogenic diet and taste delicious.)

Once you are adapted to a cyclical ketogenic diet, you can begin replacing one day a week of ketogenic eating with a KetoFast day, when you consume only 300 to 600 calories of carefully chosen foods (such as those outlined in the recipes in this book), which will keep your body in a fasted state and stimulate your body's natural healing response.

You can gradually work up to two KetoFast days per week.

PROCESS FOR ADAPTING TO KETOFASTING

Step one: Stop eating three hours before bedtime.

Step two: Begin shortening your eating window—typically this is most easily done by continuing to not eat for three hours before bedtime and then delaying breakfast.

Step three: As you gradually reduce your eating window to between six and eight hours a day, begin following a ketogenic diet.

Step four: After you are regularly producing ketones, add in one "feast" day a week when you eat more net carbs and protein in what's known as a cyclical ketogenic diet.

Step five: Add in one day of KetoFasting a week for one month (a total of four weeks).

Step six: If you are doing well and feel comfortable, progress to two days a week of KetoFasting. The other days you should still be following a cyclical ketogenic diet—four days of a strictly ketogenic diet, one day when you consume a higher level of carbs (say 50 to 100 grams) and two days of KetoFasting a week. You can continue with this strategy until you reach your health goals.

CALCULATE YOUR KETOFAST CALORIE TARGET

It is important that you don't overeat on your KetoFast days, as you want your body to have a typical physiological response to a lack of food. If you eat too much, your body won't go into a fasted state. So you want to be precise about the number of calories you consume.

The way you determine how much you should be eating on your Keto-Fast days is to subtract your body fat percentage from 100—that number is your percentage of lean body tissue. (To determine your body fat percentage, I recommend buying an electronic scale that calculates it. There are many models available online that cost about $25, although you can also use calipers or a dual-energy X-ray absorptiometry [DEXA] scan to measure it.) Then multiply your total body weight by your percentage of lean body tissue; the result is your lean body mass. Finally, multiply your lean body mass by 3.5 to arrive at the approximate number of calories you should have on your KetoFast day—it should be somewhere between 300 and 600 calories. In general, a small woman requires about 300 calories and a larger man needs closer to 600 calories.

It's best to have all your calories as one meal rather than breaking it up throughout the day. An early lunch may be ideal, as it gives you three to four hours after rising and before you go to bed to be burning fat; it also generally coincides with the time when your energy needs are highest for the rest of the day, unless you have a highly physical job, such as landscaping or carpentry, that requires you to expend a lot of physical energy early in the morning.

DETERMINE YOUR KETOFAST MACRONUTRIENT BREAKDOWN

On your partial fasting days, it's important to consider what *types* of calories you consume—not just how many. There are three main types of foods, known as macronutrients: protein, fat, and carbohydrates. You want to keep the ratio of these macronutrients in proper proportion so that you maintain ketosis and keep your fat-burning high. That means you will want to keep both your carbohydrate and protein intake below 15 to 20 grams each. If the calories from these two categories of foods don't add up to your targeted intake, add the remaining calories as fat, typically in the form of coconut oil or MCT/C8 oil. To help you keep track of your macronutrient intake, I suggest you use Cronometer—a food tracking tool that I discuss on page 29—to input the food you plan to eat on your KetoFast day *before* you have eaten it, so you can see how much additional fat you'll need to take to meet your caloric total.

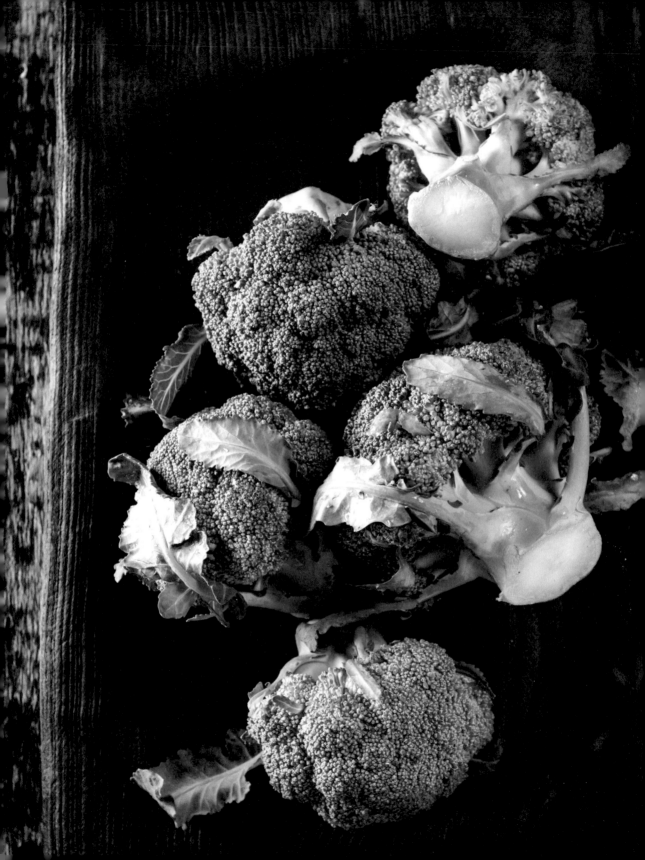

Cruciferous vegetables are a fundamental part of the KetoFast plan. These veggies—including broccoli, cabbage, collards, brussels sprouts, cauliflower, kale, and bok choy, to name just a few—have been repeatedly shown to be some of nature's most valuable health-promoting foods, capable of preventing a number of common health issues.

Because they are low-carb, nutrient-rich, and chock-full of compounds that help promote detox (among other benefits, which I'll enumerate here), they are the mainstay of many of the KetoFast-friendly recipes in this book, and also deserve a large presence on your plate when you are following a cyclical ketogenic diet.

The super-nutrients that these veggies provide include: fiber, the anticancer compounds sulforaphane[1, 2, 3, 4] and other powerful isothiocyanates,[5, 6] anti-inflammatory and free radical quenching phenolic compounds,[7, 8, 9] and immune-boosting diindolylmethane (DIM).[10, 11]

In addition, compounds found in broccoli and other cruciferous veggies have been shown to:[12]

- **Reduce the risk of obesity.**
- **Suppress chronic inflammation,** in part by reducing (by as much as 73 percent) reactive oxygen species that cause cell damage,[13] and in part through the creation of short-chain fatty acids (SCFAs), which have been shown to lessen your risk of inflammatory diseases.[14]
- **Support healthy liver function** by improving gene expression in your liver, and lower your risk of nonalcoholic fatty liver disease.
- **Improve blood pressure** in those with hypertension.[15]
- **Reduce the risk of osteoarthritis,**[16, 17] in part by blocking enzymes linked to joint destruction.
- **Improve type 2 diabetes** by reducing glucose production. In one study, patients with dysregulated diabetes who received broccoli sprout extract in

addition to metformin had 10 percent lower fasting blood glucose levels than the placebo group.[18] Sulforaphane also lowers your risk of other health problems associated with type 2 diabetes, such as heart disease and stroke.[19, 20]

- **Improve kidney function and prevent kidney disease** by normalizing DNA methylation. DNA methylation[21] is the process by which a methyl group is added to part of a DNA molecule, which suppresses viral- and other disease-related gene expression. DNA methylation plays a role in a number of aspects of health, including hypertension, kidney function,[22] gut health,[23] and cancer.

- **Improve allergies and asthma** by reducing oxidative stress in your airways and countering cell damage caused by pollution and allergens.[24]

- **Aid in the treatment of colitis and leaky gut.**[25, 26, 27, 28]

- **Protect against neurodegenerative diseases** such as Parkinson's and Alzheimer's disease[29]

- **Promote healthy, beautiful skin** (a side effect of improved liver function and detox).

As if that list of benefits isn't enough to entice you to eat more cruciferous vegetables, another of their important health benefits is their heart-healthy influence: they lower your risk of stroke and heart attack by promoting more supple neck arteries and preventing the buildup of arterial plaque.

One study[30] that examined the effects of vegetable intake on carotid artery measures, which are indicative of arterial health (as narrow, hard arteries restrict blood flow and can lead to heart attack and stroke), found those who consumed the most cruciferous vegetables had thinner and therefore healthier carotid arteries than those who consumed the fewest.

On average, those who ate at least three daily servings of cruciferous veggies had carotid arterial walls (the artery in your neck) nearly 0.05 millimeters thinner than those who ate two servings or less. Each 0.1-millimeter decrease in thickness is associated with a decreased stroke and heart attack risk ranging from 10 to 18 percent, so the results were considered rather significant.

Overall, each 10-gram daily serving of cruciferous vegetables was associated with a 0.8 percent reduction in carotid artery wall thickness. This link was not found with other types of vegetables.

Let's take a look at some of the specific compounds that make cruciferous vegetables so potent:

Nicotinamide adenine dinucleotide (NAD+). A basic premise of aging is that your cells' ability to produce energy declines with age. With less available NAD+ coenzyme support, your cell repair and maintenance declines as well, and with that, degeneration sets in. Cruciferous vegetables have been shown to slow age-related decline in health by restoring metabolism to more youthful levels.[31, 32, 33] At least part of the mechanism by which they do that is through the coenzyme family of NAD, a compound involved in mitochondrial health and energy metabolism. NAD+ is vital for mitochondrial functionality.[34] NAD+ is also required to regenerate glutathione, necessary to prevent and minimize cellular damage due to oxidative stresses from metabolizing food or external toxic exposures.[35]

Research[36] has shown that when NAD+ synthesis in fat tissue is defective, metabolic dysfunction occurs throughout your entire body, including your skeletal muscle, heart, and liver. When NAD+ levels were restored, all of these dysfunctions were reversed. So by improving your NAD+ status, you'll improve your overall metabolism and mitochondrial health, which benefits your whole body.

Indole-3-carbinol (I3C) and diindolylmethane (DIM). Another important phytochemical found in cruciferous veggies is I3C, which in your gut is converted into DIM. DIM in turn boosts immune function and plays a role in the prevention and treatment of cancer.[37, 38]

Aside from converting to DIM, which has anticancer activity, I3C also works by activating a protein called aryl hydrocarbon receptor (AhR), which communicates with immune and epithelial cells in your gut lining, thereby helping to reduce inflammation caused by pathogenic bacteria. AhR also helps stem cells convert into mucus-producing cells in your gut lining. These cells help extract nutrients from the foods you eat, all of which translates into improved gut function and health.

When you have insufficient amounts of AhR, the stem cells end up producing malfunctioning cells that divide in an uncontrolled manner. This abnormal cell division is ultimately what results in abnormal growths that can turn into malignant tumors in your colon. Consumption of cruciferous vegetables helps prevent this chain of events by boosting I3C.

Research has also shown it can help balance male and female hormones, thereby supporting reproductive health in both sexes. DIM has been shown to balance 4-hydroxyestrone, an estrogen that can have damaging effects and plays a role in reproductive cancers. In one study, supplementation with I3C at dosages of 200 and 400 milligrams per day for three months reversed early-stage cervical cancer in 8 of 17 women.[39]

Sulforaphane. Broccoli and other cruciferous vegetables are also an excellent source of sulforaphane, a powerful phytochemical. Studies have shown sulforaphane supports normal cell function and division while causing apoptosis (programmed cell death) in colon,[40] liver,[41] prostate,[42] breast,[43] and tobacco-induced lung cancer.[44] Just three servings of broccoli per week may reduce a man's risk of prostate cancer by more than 60 percent.[45] Sulforaphane-containing broccoli sprout extract also improved fasting glucose in adults with obesity and type 2 diabetes.[46]

This sulfur compound also helps normalize your DNA methylation and increases enzymes in your liver that help destroy cancer-causing chemicals you may consume or be exposed to in your environment. It is also known to block inflammation and damage to joint cartilage.[47]

Sulforaphane may also be helpful in the treatment of breast cancer. When tested in mice and cell cultures, sulforaphane was found to target and kill cancer stem cells, thereby preventing the formation and spread of tumors.[48] Researchers believe sulforaphane may also prove useful for fighting Alzheimer's disease by altering the production of amyloid beta and tau, two main factors known to contribute to Alzheimer's disease.

In Alzheimer's patients, levels of amyloid beta protein may become abnormally high, clumping together to form plaques that disrupt neuron function. Abnormal accumulations of tau protein may also collect inside neurons, forming threads, or neurofibrillary tangles, which disrupt communication between neurons.

In a mouse model of Alzheimer's disease, sulforaphane not only cleared the accumulation of amyloid beta and tau protein, but also improved memory deficits in the mice, hinting at a potential treatment that could also be useful in humans.[49]

Eating more cruciferous veggies in an attempt to boost your sulforaphane intake, or taking it via high-quality supplement, is useful for far more than brain health. For instance, sulforaphane may be helpful in the treatment of diabetes as well as lowering blood glucose levels and improving gene expression in your liver. In fact, sulforaphane was found to inhibit glucose production in cultured cells and improve glucose tolerance in rodents on high-fat or high-fructose diets. Sulforaphane-containing broccoli sprout extract also improved fasting glucose in adults with obesity and type 2 diabetes.[50]

In addition, studies have shown that sulforaphane:

- Activates nuclear factor-like 2 (Nrf2), a transcription factor that regulates cellular oxidative stress and aids in detoxification,[51] as well as other phase 2 detoxification enzymes. In one study, sulforaphane was found to increase excretion of airborne pollutants by 61 percent.[52]

- Reduces damaging reactive oxygen species (ROS) by as much as 73 percent, thereby lowering your risk of inflammation,[53] which is a hallmark of cancer. It also lowers C-reactive protein, a marker of inflammation.[54]

- Reduces the expression of long noncoding RNA in prostate cancer cells, thereby influencing the micro RNA and reducing the cancer cells' ability to form colonies by as much as 400 percent.[55]

HOW YOU PREPARE YOUR VEGGIES, AND WHAT YOU EAT THEM WITH, MATTERS

When you eat raw mature broccoli, you only get about 12 percent of the total sulforaphane content theoretically available based on the parent compound. You can increase this amount and really maximize the cancer-fighting power of broccoli by preparing it properly.

Steaming your broccoli spears for three to four minutes will optimize the sulforaphane content by eliminating epithiospecifier protein—a heat-sensitive sulfur-grabbing protein that inactivates sulforaphane—while still retaining the enzyme myrosinase,[56] which converts glucoraphanin to sulforaphane. Without it, you cannot get any sulforaphane.

If you opt for boiling, blanch the broccoli in boiling water for no more than 20 to 30 seconds, then immerse it in cold water to stop the cooking process. Boiling or microwaving your broccoli past the one-minute mark is NOT recommended, as it will destroy a majority of the myrosinase and you will not be able to convert the glucoraphanin to sulforaphane.

You can further augment the perks of consuming sulforaphane-rich vegetables by pairing them with a myrosinase-containing food.[57] Myrosinase is an enzyme that converts glucoraphanin to sulforaphane. Examples of foods containing myrosinase include mustard seed, daikon radishes, wasabi, arugula, and coleslaw, with mustard seed being the most potent.

LIQUIDS ACCEPTABLE FOR KETOFASTING DAYS

Just as your food choices on your fasting days can support your detoxing efforts, so can the things you drink. And, of course, you'll want to avoid any beverages with artificial ingredients (such as diet sodas, sports drinks, and many enhanced waters) and/or sugars (including fruit juices and sodas).

- Water, unlimited
- Herbal tea, unlimited but choose from organic and naturally detoxifying teas, including rooibos, honeybush, dandelion root, and chamomile
- Coffee, up to six cups a day, hot or iced, must be organic
- Homemade bone broth, as long as it does not cause you to exceed your target caloric intake

What You Can Add to Your Water

- Lime slices (don't consume the limes)
- Lemon slices (don't consume the lemons)
- Apple cider vinegar (raw, organic, with "the mother"—the culture of beneficial bacteria that converts regular apple cider into vinegar)
- Celtic, Redmond, or Himalayan salt

What You Can Add to Your Coffee or Tea (Up to 1 Tablespoon)

- Coconut oil
- MCT/C8 oil (Ketone Energy)
- Butter (organic, pastured, preferably raw)
- Ghee (organic, pastured)
- Heavy cream (organic, pastured, preferably raw)
- Ground cinnamon
- Lemon (for tea or water)

Why Herbal Teas Are a Great Choice to Support Detox

I carefully selected the teas I recommend you drink on your KetoFast days because each will help your body process

and/or eliminate toxins, reduce inflammation, and, in the case of chamomile, get the rest you need to allow your body to do its important detoxification work. Below is a bit more about the unique benefits of each.

Rooibos: Also known as red tea or red bush tea, rooibos is an herbal tea that's derived from the *Aspalathus linearis* plant, a bush native to the mountainous region of Cederberg in South Africa. Rooibos contains aspalathin and quercetin, which are powerful antioxidants that can help protect the cells against damage caused by free radicals. Rooibos tea is naturally caffeine-free, and has a mildly sweet, nutty taste.

Honeybush: This medicinal tea is made from the *Cyclopia intermedia* plant that is native to the cape of South Africa. Honeybush tea is high in antioxidant phenolic compounds that are effective in reducing inflammation. Traditionally it has been used to relieve colds and other viral infections. It has also been found to significantly protect against the mutation of DNA in the liver in the presence of toxins.[58]

Dandelion root: Some people think that dandelion is nothing but a pesky weed that can ruin a perfectly groomed lawn or garden, while others consider it one of the most useful gifts from nature. It's true that dandelion may not always grow in the desired location, but this resilient plant has plenty of health benefits to offer. Tea made from dandelion roots is known for its ability to help stimulate the appetite and relieve liver and gallbladder problems. Dandelion tea is considered a "liver tonic," since it helps detoxify the liver and improve the flow of bile.

A 2017 study showed that the water-soluble polysaccharides from dandelion root may help protect the liver from hepatic injury.[59] Dandelion tea may also help improve the health of your kidneys and reduce your risk of developing gallstones by flushing out toxins, salt, and excess water through increased urine production.[60]

In addition to the benefits mentioned above, drinking roasted dandelion root tea may be beneficial for coffee lovers who are trying to cut down their caffeine intake, as it tastes relatively similar to coffee but provides better health benefits.

Chamomile: This is one of the most soothing of all herbal teas—with a long history of beneficial use dating back to ancient Egypt. Chamomile is the common name for several daisy-like plants belonging to the Asteraceae family, namely German chamomile (*Matricaria retutica*) and Roman or English chamomile (*Chamaemelum nobile*).

Chamomile has long been used to treat insomnia and is highly regarded for its ability to induce daytime calmness and relaxation. Its sedative effects are likely due to the flavonoid apigenin, which binds to benzodiazepine receptors in your brain.

Chamomile is also particularly helpful in dispelling gas, soothing heartburn, and relaxing muscles that move food through your intestines. It also inhibits *Helicobacter pylori*, a bacterium linked to stomach ulcers.

The reason that I make it a point to drink a cup of chamomile tea most nights is that it is relatively high in a flavone (a class of flavonoid that is a component of white or yellow pigments) called apigenin, which just happens to inhibit CD38. And when you inhibit CD38, you will increase NAD+ levels. NAD+ is a compound involved in mitochondrial health and whole-body metabolism—including your skeletal muscle, heart, and liver—that declines with age. The take-home message here is that by improving your NAD+ status, you'll improve your overall metabolism and mitochondrial health, which benefits your whole body.

Other Useful Teas and Herbs

The cytochrome P450 enzymes (CYP) are a superfamily of enzymes important for the metabolism of toxins. High concentrations of CYPs are mostly found in the liver, but also in your small and large intestine, lungs, and brain. The expression and activity of CYP in your liver can be increased or decreased by bioactive compounds from plants.[61] This is one of the reasons you want to avoid grapefruit juice, as it has been shown to inhibit CYP activity and lower toxin removal.[62] Studies show that St. John's wort, common valerian, Ginkgo biloba, and common sage can increase CYP activity and may be useful on partial fasting days.[63] Chicory has also been shown to increase CYP activity.[64]

UP YOUR NUTRITION WITHOUT A LOT OF CALORIES BY EATING SEEDS

Seeds are truly a miracle of nature as they contain all the nutrition needed to create and nurture a new plant. When you choose the right types, they nourish your cells, tissues, and organs with omega-3 fats, fiber, minerals, antioxidants, and other substances unique to seeds. As such, they are a powerful way to sustain you on your KetoFast days, as well as an excellent addition to your diet on all other days.

It is best to activate the sprouting process before consuming seeds, though, as this will inactivate some of the antinutrients that are present in seeds, which could limit their effectiveness. So the minimum that you would want to soak your seeds would be for 8 to 12 hours.

You could eat them after that soaking process, but I believe it is even better to take the sprouting process further and put them in wide-mouth Mason jars, rinse them twice a day, and let them drain. You can do this for up to five days, by which time most of the seeds will be sprouted and can be put into a smoothie. Alternatively, you could toss them into your salad.

Black cumin seeds

Black cumin, also known as black seed, black caraway, onion seed, and Roman coriander, is not the same as cumin. Black cumin comes from the flowering plant *Nigella sativa*, and its name in Old Latin, *panacea*, means "cure all." This powerful seed protects a wide spectrum of the body systems that participate in the detox process, including the kidneys, the liver, the GI tract, and the immune system.[65] Black cumin may also have anti-obesity effects, including contributing to reductions in body weight and waist and hip circumference.[66]

While I particularly like black cumin seeds for their healthy balance of omega-3 and omega-6 fats, I also am keenly interested in their thymoquinone content, which is known to have anticancer effects.[67] Research has recently shown that this unique substance and its derivatives are potent antioxidants that *target* mitochondria—that is, they penetrate cell membranes and accumulate in the cells' mitochondria where they're able to scavenge destructive reactive oxygen species (ROS) and free radicals.

A popular ingredient in North Indian, Pakistani, and Iranian cuisines, black cumin's taste is described as "warm and slightly bitter," resembling a blend of thyme, oregano, and nutmeg. I add a small scoop of black cumin seeds to my smoothie each day. They can be sprinkled over a salad or added to casseroles, stir-fries, salad dressings, and baked goods. Try mixing them with lemon, chopped cilantro, and tahini for a delicious topping or dip for fresh vegetables.

Black cumin can be made into a hot soothing beverage: Pour hot water over a tablespoon of seeds and steep for 10 minutes for a rejuvenating cup of tea.

You can even add a few seeds to your favorite tea or coffee for an exotic kick!

Black sesame seeds

Black sesame seeds have the highest oil content of any seed; oil comprises 50 percent of their weight, and much of that oil is made up of omega-3 fats. Many people take the extracted oil as a supplement, but I believe the whole unprocessed seeds offer more potential benefits.

Unlike white sesame seeds, black sesame seeds are unhulled, giving them a more complex flavor and additional nutritional benefits. Black sesame seeds have more calcium per gram than any other food and are excellent sources of magnesium, copper, and zinc. Like flax, they are also rich in lignans—plant compounds that act like antioxidants and are important for cellular and mitochondrial health. Once ingested, lignans are converted into weak forms of estrogen that help regulate hormone balance in the body, and could potentially help reduce the risk of hormone-associated cancers (breast, uterine, ovarian, and prostate). There is also research suggesting that postmenopausal women who have a high intake of dietary lignans have a 17 percent lower risk of breast cancer compared to those with a low intake.[68]

Flaxseeds

Flaxseeds are small, brown-colored seeds that are a source of alpha-linolenic acid (ALA), a plant-based essential omega-3 short-chain fat that your body can't make.

Not only do flaxseeds contain higher levels of omega-3s than any other plant food, but they also have a *higher ratio* of omega-3 to omega-6 fats, which is very important to your health. They're also the best source of lignans of any food. Lignans, as discussed in the black sesame seed entry, are insoluble fibers and polyphenols that your body converts into weak forms of phytoestrogens.

That may sound as if eating flaxseeds might disrupt hormonal balance, but it actually promotes stasis as lignans block the enzyme involved in estrogen production and take up space on estrogen receptor sites, which means that stronger estrogens, either manufactured in the body or taken up from the environment, aren't taken up by these receptors. Since breast cancer is associated with high levels of estrogen, this makes flaxseeds protective against breast cancer, as well as prostate and colon cancer. Flaxseeds are also traditionally used to regulate the menstrual cycle and reduce symptoms of PMS and menopause. Flaxseeds provide substantially more lignans than sesame seeds—approximately 10 times the amount.

And flaxseeds are treasure troves for fiber, both soluble and insoluble. In fact, 95 percent of flaxseed is fiber! Like other high-soluble-fiber foods, when you eat flaxseeds, they turn into a thick, gel-like mass, thanks to their high lignan levels. This "mucilage" gel serves multiple purposes. It can help increase nutrient absorption by delaying the emptying of your food into the small intestine. In turn, this helps you feel fuller longer, and helps reduce your cravings for carbs and sugar.

Whole flaxseeds should be freshly ground (in an inexpensive coffee or spice grinder) just prior to eating, and both the whole and ground seeds should be stored in the freezer or refrigerator to keep them fresh. (If they develop a rancid odor, toss them out and purchase more.) An important caution here is to avoid using preground flaxseeds or even worse, flaxseed oil, which is virtually guaranteed to be highly oxidized and rancid.

But the best way to consume flax is not to grind it at all but to soak 1 tablespoon of the flaxseeds overnight in water and then pour it into your smoothie. Alternatively, you could sprout the flaxseeds over a few days and put that into your smoothie.

Hemp seeds

Hemp seeds, or hemp hearts (the hulled seeds), have endured a bad rap for many years, largely because of their association with marijuana, or cannabis. While hemp is a variety of the cannabis plant, it is not a source of tetrahydrocannabinoids (THC)—in other words, there are no psychoactive cannabinoids, and it won't get you high.

What hemp seeds *will* do is provide an abundance of health-promoting nutrients including gamma-linolenic acid (GLA), a building block for hormone-like substances that help regulate body temperature, smooth muscle, hormone balance, and inflammation. Hemp seeds also contain abundant fiber, both insoluble

and soluble, that helps promote regularity, feeds your beneficial gut bacteria, and supports your overall digestive health. Hemp seeds contain an ideal balance of omega-3 to omega-6 fats, all 20 amino acids, manganese, vitamin E, magnesium, and phosphorus.

Chia seeds

Chia seeds, which are members of the *Salvia hispanica* family, were a prized food to the ancient Aztecs and Mayans. In fact, *chia* is the ancient Mayan word for "strength," and the tiny seeds were valued for their energy-boosting properties.

Chia seeds are a quick and easy-to-use source of protein, healthy fats, dietary fiber, minerals, vitamins, and antioxidants, all rolled into one tiny package. Although they have similar health benefits to flaxseeds, chia seeds don't have to be ground prior to consumption, and they don't go rancid as quickly either. In fact, chia seeds are said to last up to two years with no refrigeration, courtesy of the high levels of antioxidants they contain.

Their high concentration of the plant-based omega-3 fat is one of their major claims to fame. Chia seeds contain up to 40 percent of their nutrients as oil, and 60 percent of that is omega-3, a high concentration of which is alpha-linolenic acid (ALA).

Another health plus: Chia seeds contain a number of phytochemicals, including myricetin, quercetin, and kaempferol, which are known for their antioxidant, anti-inflammatory, and anticancer properties. Perhaps their greatest benefit is their high amount of fiber. Chia seeds contain about 5 grams of fiber in just 1 tablespoon.

When chia seeds are soaked in water or coconut milk overnight, they take on a tapioca-like texture; add some cinnamon and/or raw cacao powder and a bit of stevia for a pudding-like treat that can be eaten any time, even on KetoFast days (just be sure to log them on Cronometer, the food-consumption-tracking app I discuss on page 29).

On other days, you can sprinkle chia over yogurt, smoothies, or soups. Since they do absorb water and become gelatinous, if it's crunch you're after, sprinkle them on just before eating. Or, sprout your chia seeds (yes, just like with a Chia Pet) and eat these nutritional superstars in salads or on their own.

Caution: If you have a history of difficulty swallowing, or are giving chia seeds to children, take care not to eat a handful of them and then immediately drink water; they can quickly form a gel-like ball that can partially block the esophagus, requiring medical treatment to remove.

Psyllium

Psyllium husk is best known for its ability to treat constipation and is the active ingredient in Metamucil (which I am not recommending here). Psyllium husk has been shown to regulate the intestinal barrier and decrease pro-inflammatory cytokines and tight junction protein expression in the colon.[69]

Even though a tablespoon of psyllium husk has 18 calories, they are all

digestive-resistant carbs, so it adds zero carbs to your dietary targets. Many find that if they put a tablespoon of organic psyllium in a glass of water and let it form a gel, they can eat it like a porridge and it will fill their stomach and alleviate their hunger pangs.

However, it is very important to understand that most psyllium, especially the psyllium found in brand products like Metamucil, is a heavily sprayed crop, which means many common sources are contaminated with pesticides, herbicides, and fertilizers. So if you are going to use psyllium, it is absolutely imperative that you make sure it is organic. You also need to make sure it's 100 percent pure: Many supplement brands use synthetic or semi-synthetic active ingredients that do *not* contain psyllium, such as methylcellulose and calcium polycarbophil. Some brands even add sweeteners and other additives, which you should avoid.

Mitomix Seed Blend

My Organic Mitomix Seed Blend is a delicious blend of the six seeds I just covered: organic golden flaxseeds, whole-husk psyllium, hulled hemp seeds, chia seeds, black sesame seeds, and black cumin seeds. Rather than having to purchase six individual products and open them all up each day to use, I now reach for my Mitomix Seed Blend—it's simple, fast, and convenient to use.

This crunchy, slightly nutty blend can be eaten alone or as a topping to meals. You can eat it straight out of the package or blend it smooth in a coffee grinder. On

KetoFast days when you need something that doesn't take any time to prepare, you can mix 1, 2, or 3 tablespoons of the Mitomix blend with 1 or 2 tablespoons of MCT oil, depending on your target calorie intake. Be sure to measure the seed blend and the MCT oil and enter it into Cronometer; 1 tablespoon of this mixture has about the same amount of calories as a tablespoon of psyllium husks alone but has an additional 2 grams of protein, and you don't want to throw off your macronutrient targets.

On non-KetoFast days, Mitomix Seed Blend is ideal for adding to smoothies and shakes, salads, yogurt, or oatmeal. Each day I add 2 tablespoons to my breakfast smoothie. It's become one of my favorite—and certainly easiest—strategies for optimizing my mitochondrial health.

I'm proud to say that the ingredients in my Mitomix Seed Blend are certified organic, ancient, and/or heirloom varieties, grown on nearby farms using sustainable practices, and traceable to source. Of course, you can buy all the seeds separately and mix them on your own, but I think you will appreciate the convenience of having them all in one bag and I don't believe you can get higher-quality seeds anywhere else.

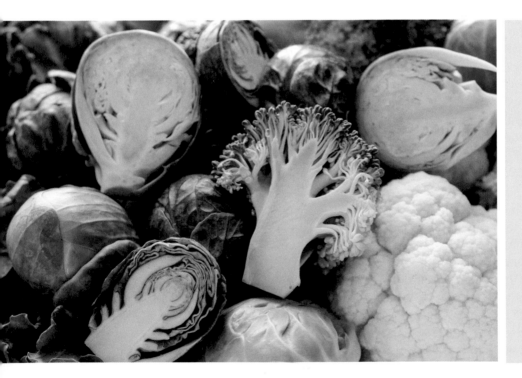

HELPFUL TOOLS AND CONSIDERATIONS

The KetoFast program is an intricate eating plan. Without an accurate recording and nutritional analysis of your food intake, it is very easy to sabotage your efforts to be successful on the program. So while it may seem like a bit of work and maybe even a little intimidating, I can assure you that you will be very glad you made the effort to record your foods.

My favorite food tracking system by far is Cronometer, which can be used on your desktop (this version is free to use) or on your mobile device (which requires a small fee to install on your phone). I like Cronometer so much, in fact, that I reached out to its founder and worked with him to customize the software to the KetoFast program. Every recipe in this cookbook that you're holding in your hands, as well as all the recipes in the *Fat for Fuel Cookbook*, have already been entered into the Cronometer database. Meaning, anytime you eat one of these recipes, you can log it at Cronometer in just one click (instead of having to add each ingredient separately). I realize that logging your food is an extra item on your to-do list, and I want to make it as simple as possible for you to do so.

It really is so enlightening and empowering to be able to objectively see everything you've eaten—how many grams of net carbs, fats, and protein you eat, as well as how much of each nutrient you are consuming and in what ratios. It makes what can feel like a fraught process—as any health-related decision or change in behavior can be—much more manageable.

HOW TO USE CRONOMETER FOR KETOFASTING

For accuracy's sake, it is important to weigh the food you eat, using an inexpensive digital kitchen scale, before you eat it.

I prefer to enter all the foods I plan to eat later that day each morning, using it like a planner. It takes the guesswork out of what I will eat and saves me some key decision-making time later in the day. It also gives you the opportunity to view that day's nutritional intake before you eat it and to add or delete foods or change portion sizes to better reach your targets.

Along these lines, it is important to point out the obvious: You need to enter every bit of food or drink that passes your lips. If you are inconsistent, or your entries don't reflect your actual portion sizes, then the data generated will be flawed and potentially damaging to your health. It is far better to be honest and record everything, even if you regret your choice as soon as you make it. That way, you can learn from experience by noting exactly how your body responded to your choice, for example, by testing your blood glucose levels after you've eaten the food that perhaps wasn't on your eating plan.

To get started, visit cronometer.com/mercola, create an account, and log in. You'll find helpful how-to videos at your first log-in. All the videos are also available for viewing at any time in the User Manual. I believe you will love the objectivity and the feedback this tool gives you and the fact that all the recipes in this cookbook are pre-entered into Cronometer so that it is as simple as possible to log the meals you eat on your partial fast days.

CONTRAINDICATIONS FOR TIME-RESTRICTED EATING AND KETOFASTING

Although most people could safely benefit from time-restricted eating and KetoFasting (once you've built up your health and your tolerance for going without food), it's important to use caution if you have certain health challenges. If any of the following situations apply to you, you should NOT participate in fasting of any kind unless approved by your physician.

- **Underweight:** Refrain from any type of fasting if you have a body mass index (BMI) of 18.5 or less.

- **Malnourished:** You need to put your focus on eating healthier, more nutritious food before you can safely do any kind of fast. I would also caution you to avoid fasting if you struggle with an eating disorder such as anorexia, even if you are not clinically underweight.

- **Young age:** Children should not fast for more than 24 hours because they need nutrients for continued growth; if your child is obese, consider cutting him or her back on refined grains and sugar to promote weight loss.

- **Pregnancy and breastfeeding:** Pregnant and breastfeeding women put their baby's healthy growth and development at risk when fasting because a consistent flow of nutrients must be shared continually with the baby to ensure its well-being.

- **Certain medications:** If you take medication and it must be taken with food to achieve the proper effect, you will need to use caution when fasting. Medications such as aspirin and metformin, as well as any other drugs that may cause stomach ulcers or stomach upset, need to be considered.

  Risks are especially high if you're on diabetic medication. If you take the same dose of medication but don't eat, you run the risk of hypoglycemia, which is when your blood sugar drops very low. This can be extremely dangerous. It's important to check with your doctor before adjusting your medication to accommodate fasting. You may need to find a doctor who has some experience with diabetes and fasting so he or she can guide you in how to implement this program safely.

- **High uric acid or a tendency toward gout:** Fasting tends to increase your uric acid level because your kidneys increase their reabsorption of uric acid when you don't eat. Most people will not experience a problem with this, but if you have gout, you may need to consult your physician before starting a fasting program.

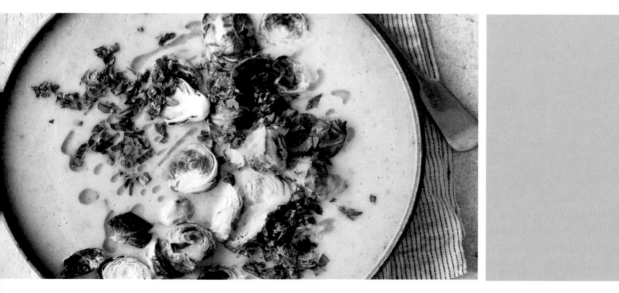

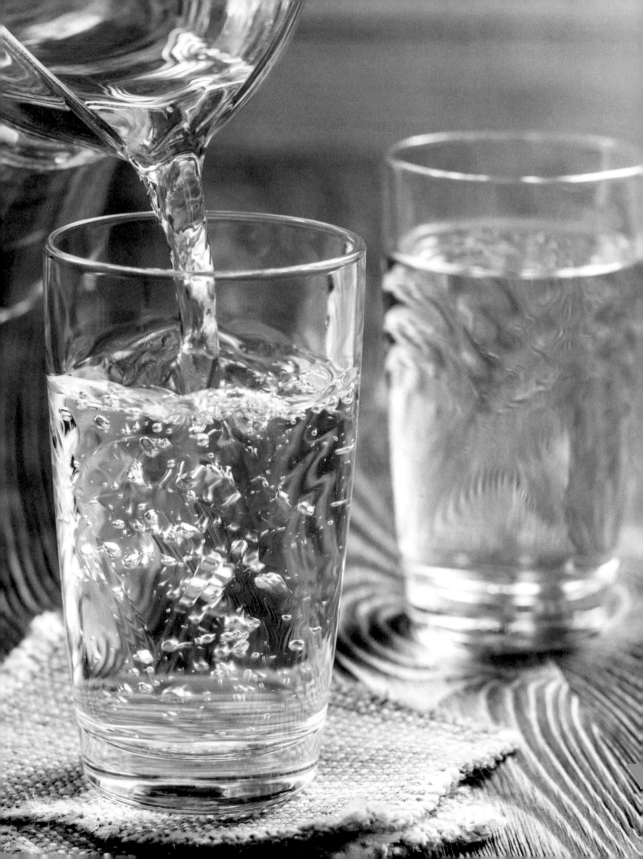

NOURISH YOUR ORGANS OF FILTRATION
Your Liver, Kidneys, and GI Tract

The process of detoxification involves moving the toxins out of your cells and into your bloodstream. Then your detox pathways that are primarily in your liver will convert these fat-soluble toxins to water-soluble toxins. Once the toxins are converted, your kidneys, skin, and gut can eliminate them, via urine, sweat, or feces.

Since we live in such a toxic world, your detoxification capacity is likely hampered. After all, every day you are likely to be exposed to a soup of different chemicals via your food, water, air, and personal-care products. Exposure to one chemical, such as glyphosate (the primary component of the ubiquitous pesticide Roundup) is bad enough—when chemicals intermingle in your body, it stands to reason that their effect is altered and intensified. A 2018 study found that when even small amounts of chemicals from food, pharmaceuticals, and personal-care products are combined in your body, you may experience liver damage.[1]

The results of this study support previous research demonstrating the effects of chemical cocktails, even at low levels,[2] on the liver.[3] To ensure your detox system is working properly, begin by supporting your kidneys, liver, and GI tract.

DRINK PLENTY OF PURE WATER

Every day, but especially on your KetoFast days, be sure to stay properly hydrated by drinking adequate amounts of pure, clean water. In my view, hydration is truly one of the foundation pillars of health, which is why I made it the very first step in my book *Effortless Healing: 9 Simple Ways to Sidestep Illness, Shed Excess Weight, and Help Your Body Fix Itself.*

Hydration becomes even more important when you are regularly engaging in partial fasting, because you need to be properly hydrated in order to detoxify and get rid of wastes through your sweat, stool, and urine. When you are partial fasting, it also becomes more important than ever to hydrate yourself with the purest, least contaminated water you can get your hands on, which is not necessarily easy as many dangerous chemicals find their way into the ecosystem, including into our water supply.

In general, it's difficult to get access to pure water in your home unless you're filtering your tap water. Most municipal water supplies contain a number of potentially hazardous contaminants at varying levels. Among the worst are disinfection by-products (DBPs). In water treatment facilities that use chlorine or chloramines to treat and purify the water, toxic DBPs form when these disinfectants react with natural organic matter like decaying vegetation in the source water.

These by-products are over 1,000 times more toxic than chlorine, and then you need to address other contaminants, such as fluoride and pharmaceutical drugs that people either urinate out or dispose of in the toilet. Trihalomethanes (THMs), among the most common DBPs, are Cancer Group B carcinogens, meaning they've been shown to cause cancer in laboratory animals. They've also been linked to reproductive problems such as spontaneous abortion, stillbirths, and congenital malformations in both animals and humans, even at lower levels of exposure. These types of DBPs may weaken your immune system, disrupt your central nervous system, damage your cardiovascular system, disrupt your renal system, and cause respiratory problems.

In a 2017 analysis by the Environmental Working Group (EWG), water samples from nearly 50,000 water utilities in 50 states revealed more than 267 different kinds of toxins in U.S. tap water.[4] Of the 267 chemicals detected:

- 93 are linked to an increased risk of cancer;
- 78 are associated with brain and nervous system damage;
- 63 are suspected of causing developmental harm to children or fetuses;
- 38 may cause fertility problems; and
- 45 are linked to hormonal disruption.

Alarmingly, nearly 19,000 public water systems had lead levels above 3.8 parts per billion, which would put a formula-fed baby at risk of elevated blood lead levels. Other chemicals of concern include:

- Chromium-6, an industrial chemical that is not regulated under the Safe Drinking Water Act but is found in drinking water in all 50 states at levels above those that may pose a cancer risk
- 1,4-dioxane, an industrial solvent that was widely detected at levels above what the Environmental Protection Agency (EPA) says could pose a cancer risk
- Nitrates, stemming from industrial agriculture, which were also found at potentially risky levels

If you have well water, it would be prudent to have your water tested for arsenic and other contaminants. If you have public water, you can get a local drinking water quality report from the EPA.[5] The agency regulates tap water in the U.S., but while there are legal limits on many of the contaminants permitted in municipal water supplies, more than half of the 300-plus chemicals detected in U.S. drinking water are unregulated, and some of the legal limits may be too lenient for safety. For a more objective view of your water quality, check out the Tap Water Database created by the EWG, available at https://www.ewg.org/tapwater/.

I recently requested a water analysis from my local water authority. First they sent a five-page PDF with measurements of four contaminants, one of which was fluoride. I then asked for the full analysis, which resulted in my receiving a 60-page report that included literally hundreds of chemicals, including 2,4-D, dioxin, and glyphosate at 4,200 parts per trillion. Unfortunately, there's no guarantee bottled water will be much better.

Aside from the issues of plastic pollution, microplastic contamination, and the problem with plastic chemicals leaching into the water, bottled water is often just as contaminated with chemicals as your tap water. Rarely does bottled water undergo superior filtration, and bottled water regulations are actually laxer than those for municipal tap water.

CHOOSING A WATER FILTRATION SYSTEM

Unless you can verify the purity of your water, seriously consider installing a high-quality, whole-house water filtration system. Ideally, filter the water both at the point of entry and at the point of use. This means filtering all the water that comes into the house, and then filtering it again at the kitchen sink and shower. As for the type of filtration system to get, there are a variety of options, most of which have both benefits and drawbacks. Here are a few of the most common options:

- **Reverse osmosis (RO):** In addition to removing chlorine and inorganic and organic contaminants in your water, RO will also remove about 80 percent of fluoride and most DPBs. Drawbacks include the need for frequent cleaning to avoid bacterial growth. Your best alternative is to use a tankless RO system with a compressor. This is because the plastic in the tank link serves as a fuel for many bacteria that quickly contaminate the tank. If you are using a tank on your RO system, it is wise to drain your tank completely dry every other day to limit this problem. The expense is another factor, as you may need the assistance of a plumber to get the system up and running. RO will also remove many valuable minerals and trace elements along with harmful contaminants.

- **Ion exchange:** Ion exchange is designed to remove dissolved salts in the water, such as calcium. This system also softens the water and helps prevent the creation of scale buildup. The ion exchange system was originally used in boilers and other industrial situations before becoming popular in home purifying units, which usually combine the system with carbon for greater effectiveness.

  While advantages include a high flow rate and low maintenance cost, science points out the disadvantages, which include calcium sulfate fouling, iron fouling, and contamination from organic matter, bacteria, and chlorine.[6]

- **Granular carbon and carbon block filters:** These are the most common types of countertop and under-counter water filters. Granular activated carbon is recognized by the EPA as the best available technology for the removal of organic chemicals like herbicides, pesticides, and industrial chemicals. One of its downfalls is that the loose material inside can channel, meaning the water creates pathways through the carbon material, thereby escaping filtering.

  Carbon block filters offer the same superior filtering ability but are compressed with the carbon medium in a solid form. This eliminates channeling and gives the ability to precisely combine multiple media in a sub-micron filter cartridge. By combining different media, the ability to selectively remove a wide range of contaminants can be achieved.

Another alternative is to collect water from natural, deep springs. There's a website called Find A Spring (findaspring.com) where you can look up natural springs in your area. Do your homework before setting off to collect water, however, as you may not be allowed to collect water from all springs, even if they're listed. None of the springs in Florida, for example, are set up to be legally used as sources of potable water. You may also want to check and see if there have been any chemical spills in the area that might affect the purity of the water. A work-around can be to check whether your local state park has a potable well you can use, as they typically draw water from the same sources as the springs.

A key component of proper hydration is getting the water into your cells. One of the simplest ways of getting water into your body is to eat more foods that contain water, such as leafy green plant foods.

In his book *The Fourth Phase of Water*, Gerald Pollack, Ph.D., reveals the importance of structured water or H_3O_2 (as opposed to H_2O, which is regular water). This structured water, also known as exclusion zone or EZ water, has unique properties. It's more viscous, dense, and alkaline than regular water; has a negative charge; and can hold and deliver energy much like a battery. In fact, this is the kind of water found in your cells, and it helps recharge your mitochondria. Two simple ways to structure your water are:

- cooling the water to 39 degrees F (about 10 degrees C); and

- creating a vortex in the water by stirring it with a spoon.

The best way to get structured water is to activate the water already inside your body by exposing your bare skin to near-infrared and ultraviolet (UV) radiation, i.e., sunlight, on a regular basis. You probably already know that sunlight can help you manufacture vitamin D, but we are beginning to understand that humans are more like plants than we ever realized. We draw energy from the sun that benefits us in multiple ways, including in how hydrated we are.

It will also be important to be certain you are getting enough salt. Many people are fearful that excess salt will increase their blood pressure or cause other problems. But in reality many are not getting enough salt, especially those who are using a sauna or doing partial fasting, as they tend to eliminate quite a bit of salt.

Just make sure that it is not commercial salt that is highly processed. Also, it has recently become clear that many sea salts are now contaminated with micro plastics from ocean plastic pollution. The book *The Salt Fix* by James DiNicolantonio, Pharm.D., is an excellent resource to get you up to speed on this topic.

If you are dehydrated at the cellular level—and most of us are, particularly if we are facing any level of illness—you won't be able to reduce your toxin accumulation effectively. So make sure you ingest enough structured water. By drinking structured water, eating green vegetables, and soaking and eating seeds, you will support your body's detoxification efforts.

MAKE BONE BROTH A REGULAR PART OF YOUR DIET

Due to its medicinal properties, bone broth is one of the foods I highly recommend, and personally use, to maintain a healthy connective tissue, as it is loaded with amino acids like glycine, proline, and hydrocyproline that strengthen your tendons and skin.

While restaurants and storefronts dedicated to serving broth have popped up in New York[7, 8] and Los Angeles[9] in recent years, the influence of bone broth on health and disease is nothing new. Well before it was elevated to a trendy health drink by elite professional athletes such as NBA star LeBron James and retired NBA icon Kobe Bryant,[10] bone broth has been recognized across cultures and for millennia for its curative properties.

In earlier generations, when it was unthinkable to waste any part of an animal carcass, resourceful hunters and cooks mastered the art of simmering otherwise unusable cartilage, bones, hooves, and skin to produce a hearty broth. In some ways, we are now rediscovering many of the antidotes and home remedies that served our grandparents and great-grandparents well just a few generations ago.

Bone broth is exactly what it sounds like: broth made from animal bones. Homemade broth differs substantially from the canned, store-bought variety or the kind produced by adding boiling water to chemical-laden bouillon cubes. In its simplest form, bone broth is made using bones, vinegar, and spices. It is simmered in a pot or slow cooker at least overnight, or as long as 72 hours. Longer simmering times result in a more complete release of gelatin, minerals, and other nutrients from the bones, which is key to realizing the many health-giving benefits and restorative properties this broth has to offer. The process of making bone broth extracts the numerous minerals that comprise the bones, including calcium, phosphorus, potassium, magnesium, and sodium. Many of these are electrolytes, which means they help improve your overall hydration and can combat some of the detox symptoms that you may experience while fasting.

The most convenient way to obtain all the benefits of bone broth is to purchase it. However, you need to be very careful about selecting products. The dirty little secret of the bone broth industry is that many of the leading brands are using animals grown in concentrated animal feeding operations (CAFO) in China that are loaded with toxins.

While you can make it yourself, it is a very long process that might be daunting for some. If you decide to make your own, you will need to identify a source for high-quality bones; the rest of the process is fairly easy and requires only a little planning. The most efficient way to create your broth is to use a slow cooker or Crock-Pot. This will allow you to put a few basic ingredients in the pot in the morning, turn it on low heat, and walk away. Come evening, you will be welcomed home by a tantalizing aroma.

You can use beef, chicken, fish, or pork bones to make your broth. You will find that each variety offers unique flavors and nutritional benefits. The most important aspect of the broth-making process is to ensure you're getting the best-quality bones that you possibly can. Ideally, you'll want to use only bones from organically raised, pastured, or grass-fed animals. Using bones from animals raised in CAFOs means your broth will lack many of the most nourishing ingredients. Besides that, CAFO animals are often fed an unnatural genetically engineered diet and frequently are given antibiotics and growth hormones. You don't want any of those potentially harmful additives in your broth, so make sure to start off with an organically raised product.

To find a local source for organic bones, connect with possible suppliers at local food co-ops, health-food stores, and farmers' markets. Many farmers love to talk about their operations, and most will be more than happy to give you the details about the feed they use and how they care for their animals. Keep in mind that very often farmers from smaller farms raise their livestock according to organic principles even if their operation has not been certified organic. This is mainly due to the reality that the certification process is quite rigorous and costly, and generally unachievable for many small farms.

You'll also want to use filtered water to make your broth.

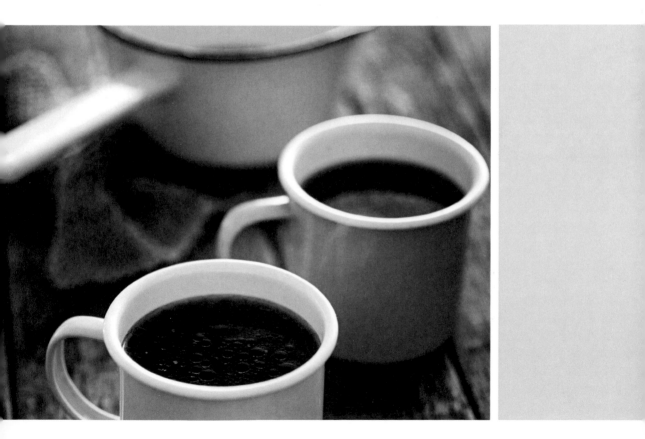

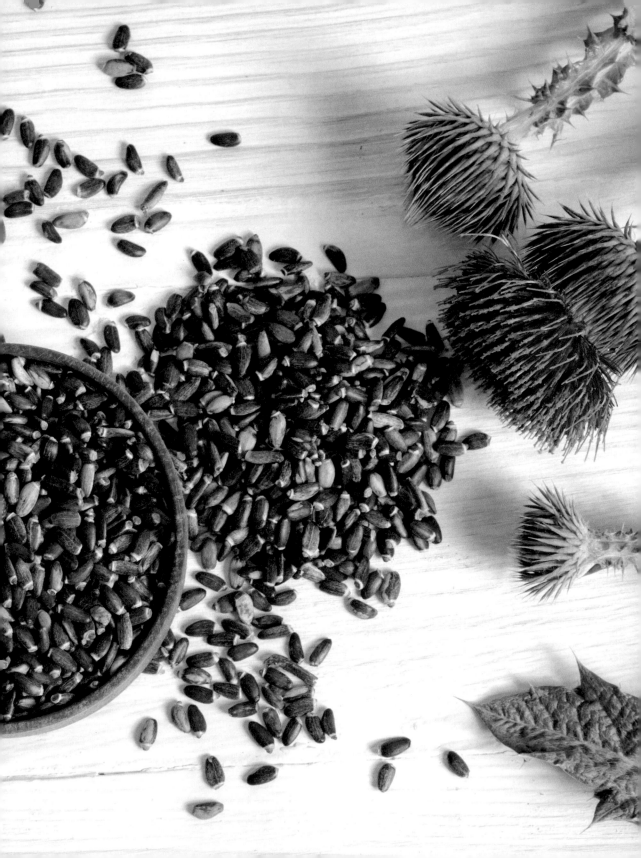

I am very conservative about recommending supplements, as I believe you're best off getting your nutrients from healthy, whole organic foods. But I'm also pragmatic, and I understand a perfect diet is hard to come by these days, so some supplements I believe can be quite beneficial in promoting detoxification.

When you have worked your way up to one or, eventually, two days a week of partial fasting, the following supplements will help your body complete the detoxification process and minimize any damaging effects from the toxins that may get liberated from your fat stores. They should be taken on days you are KetoFasting.

Ubiquinol (the reduced form of CoQ10): 100 to 150 milligrams twice a day. Coenzyme Q is necessary for your mitochondrial energy production and regulates the expression of genes that are important for inflammatory processes, growth, and detoxification reactions.[1]

Organic whole psyllium husks: 1 to 2 tablespoons. Psyllium is an excellent source of both soluble and insoluble fiber, which means it will add bulk to your stool and help your body excrete more of the toxins that make it to the GI tract. As psyllium contains about 18 calories per

tablespoon, be sure to add this into your Cronometer data so you will hit your appropriate calorie target. For more information on psyllium, please see page 27.

High-quality probiotics: Follow dosage guidelines on the packaging. Look for one with *L. rhamnosus*, which has been shown to reduce pesticide toxicity,[2] and *L. plantarum*, which has been shown to reduce the negative effects of mycotoxin exposure.[3] The Complete Probiotics that I sell on mercola.com is an excellent source of these and other useful strains, but there are other companies that sell probiotics that contain these strains. Just make sure that whatever probiotic supplement you choose is high potency.

Magnesium: Magnesium is the fourth-most abundant mineral in your body and is involved in more than 600 different biochemical reactions. It facilitates all of your body's enzymatic processes, including detoxification. Magnesium is also important for brain health, cellular health and function, and the optimization of your mitochondria. And up to 80 percent of people are estimated to be deficient in magnesium.

Magnesium resides at the center of the chlorophyll molecule, so if you rarely eat fresh leafy greens, you're probably not getting much magnesium from your diet. Furthermore, while eating organic whole foods will help optimize your magnesium intake, it's still not a surefire way to ward off magnesium deficiency, as most soils have become severely depleted of nutrients, including magnesium.

Magnesium absorption is also dependent on having sufficient amounts of selenium, parathyroid hormone, and vitamins B6 and D and is hindered by excess ethanol, salt, coffee, and phosphoric acid in soda. Stress, lack of sleep, excessive menstruation, and certain drugs (especially diuretics and proton-pump inhibitors) also deplete your body of magnesium.[4] For these reasons, many experts recommend taking supplemental magnesium.

The recommended daily allowance (RDA) for magnesium is around 310 to 420 milligrams per day depending on your age and sex,[5] but many experts believe you may need 600 to 900 milligrams per day, which is more in line with the magnesium uptake during the Paleolithic period. Personally, I believe many may benefit from amounts as high as 1 to 2 grams (1,000 to 2,000 milligrams) of elemental magnesium per day. Most of us have high chemical and electromagnetic field (EMF) exposures, and the extra magnesium should help lower the associated damage. *Elemental* refers to how much pure magnesium is in each milligram, or what percent is actual magnesium.

One of the best forms is magnesium threonate, as it appears to be the most efficient at penetrating cell membranes, including your mitochondria and blood-brain barrier. If your body agrees with the higher doses of magnesium, it is best to take it in evenly divided doses throughout the day to prevent loose stools. It can be taken with or without food. If you're also taking calcium, take them together.

While the ideal ratio of magnesium to calcium is thought to be 1-to-1, most people get far more calcium than magnesium from their diet; hence, your need for supplemental magnesium may be two to three times greater than calcium.

Milk thistle: The milk thistle herb has been used for thousands of years to support liver, kidney, and gallbladder health. The herb is native to the Mediterranean and is regarded as a weed in some areas of the world. When the leaves are crushed, they release a milky sap, which is where the herb gets its characteristic name.

Silymarin is a group of flavonoids (silibinin, silidianin, and silicristin) known to help repair your liver cells when they've been damaged by toxic substances. These flavonoids also protect new liver cells from being destroyed by toxins. As such, milk thistle greatly improves the overall functioning of your liver, with specific applications related to cirrhosis of the liver, chronic liver inflammation, and liver damage from alcohol and other intoxicating substances.

Milk thistle is available in a capsule, extract, or powder form shown to benefit your liver, gallbladder, heart, and prostate. According to the National Institutes of Health, silymarin is the most commonly used herbal supplement in the U.S. for liver problems.[6] It is also useful as an essential oil.

You can find milk thistle at most health food stores under the names silymarin or silybum. Your best options are extracts of milk thistle with silybum or silymarin standardized to 70 to 80 percent. The recommended daily intake is 420 milligrams in divided doses. While you can stay on milk thistle indefinitely, it is not generally recommended. Be sure to consult with your doctor before taking milk thistle on a continuing basis, especially if you are using other medications.

NAC: N-acetylcysteine (NAC) is an incredibly useful supplement that has many benefits related to its ability to boost production of glutathione, an antioxidant that is used to reduce free radical damage and that plays a role in the detoxification of heavy metals and other harmful substances.

The most common use of NAC is for liver support, especially to counteract the effects of alcohol and acetaminophen, two common compounds metabolized through the liver and associated with liver damage.

NAC supplementation can help "pre-tox" your body when taken before alcohol, thereby minimizing the damage associated with alcohol consumption. NAC is a form of the amino acid cysteine, which, in addition to increasing glutathione, also reduces the acetaldehyde toxicity that causes many hangover symptoms. Taking NAC (at least 200 milligrams) 30 minutes before you drink can help lessen the alcohol's toxic effects.[7] It is thought to work even better when combined with vitamin B_1 (thiamine).[8] All of that said, it's important to realize that this protocol will not reduce your susceptibility to alcohol poisoning or other acute adverse events associated with binge drinking, so please use common sense and drink responsibly. NAC is also used as an antidote for

acetaminophen toxicity, which also causes liver damage by depleting glutathione.

NAC is widely available as an oral dietary supplement and is relatively inexpensive. Considering its wide array of health benefits, it's a supplement worthy of consideration for many. Unfortunately, it's rather poorly absorbed when taken orally. According to some studies,[9, 10] oral bioavailability may range between 4 and 10 percent. Its half-life is also in the neighborhood of two hours, which is why most study subjects take it two or three times a day.

Due to its poor bioavailability, the recommended dosage can go as high as 1,800 milligrams per day. No maximum safe dose has yet been determined, but as a general rule, it's well-tolerated and has no known serious side effects, although some do experience gastrointestinal side effects such as nausea, diarrhea, or constipation. Should this occur, reduce your dosage. It's also best taken in combination with food, to reduce the likelihood of gastrointestinal effects.

Since NAC boosts glutathione, which is a powerful detox agent, you may experience debilitating detox symptoms if you start with too high a dose. To avoid this, start low, with say 400 to 600 milligrams once a day, and work your way up. Also, if you are currently taking an antidepressant or undergoing cancer treatment, be sure to discuss the use of NAC with your physician, as it may interact with some antidepressants and chemotherapy.

MSM: Methylsulfonylmethane (MSM) is the first oxidized metabolite of dimethyl sulfoxide (DMSO)[11] and a naturally occurring sulfur compound found in all vertebrates. When you have insufficient MSM your cells become hard and stiff, which means they can't allow for adequate flushing of foreign particles and free radicals.[12]

As a supplement, MSM is widely used in the treatment of pain, especially pain associated with arthritic conditions. One clinical trial found that people with osteoarthritis of the knee who took 3 grams of MSM twice a day for 12 weeks experienced significantly decreased pain and improved physical function, compared to a placebo.[13]

MSM is 34 percent sulfur by weight. Sulfur has only recently become more widely appreciated as a critical nutrient, without which many other things don't work properly. If you don't have enough sulfur in your system, you're not going to be able to naturally produce the most important antioxidant that your body produces: glutathione, which is absolutely essential for removing heavy metals and many of the toxins you're exposed to. Without sulfur, glutathione cannot work.

As a supplement, most tolerate up to 4 grams daily with few known and mild side effects.[14] Clinical research studies have found the effective amounts range from about 1.5 grams to 6 grams.

That said, potential side effects at higher doses include intestinal discomfort, ankle swelling, and skin rashes. These are likely detoxifying effects that can typically be mitigated or minimized by cutting back on the initial dosage and slowly working your way up.

It's a bit of a challenge to get an ample amount of sulfur from your diet these days. There's been a transition away from many foods that have traditionally been big sources of sulfur, like collagen or keratin. If you make bone broth—by cooking down bones from organically raised animals—and drink it regularly (or use it for soups and stews), that definitely helps. The connective tissues are sulfur-rich, and when you slow-cook the bones, you dissolve these nutrients out of the bone and into the water.

DIM: Indole-3-carbinol (I3C) is a potent phytochemical found in cruciferous vegetables like broccoli, brussel sprouts, cabbage, and cauliflower. Once eaten, your gut converts I3C into diindolylmethane (DIM). DIM in turn boosts immune function, plays a role in the prevention and treatment of cancer,[15, 16] and acts as a powerful antioxidant.

DIM also has other health benefits. Research has shown that it can help balance male and female hormones, thereby supporting reproductive health in both sexes. Importantly, DIM has been shown to balance 4-hydroxyestrone, an estrogen that can have damaging effects and plays a role in reproductive cancers. In one study, supplementation with I3C at dosages of 200 and 400 milligrams per day for three months reversed early-stage cervical cancer in 8 of 17 women.[17]

It also supports your liver's detoxification processes, and helps heal liver damage by supporting the reproduction of normal, healthy cells. If you are taking the seeds as mentioned previously, you likely will not need this supplement as it is in the seeds naturally.

Broccoli seed extract or broccoli sprout powder: These two supplements are excellent sources of I3C and DIM; they also have the extra benefit of providing other compounds found in broccoli that a DIM supplement can't: glucoraphanin and the enzyme myrosinase, which is required to convert glucoraphanin to sulforaphane. Sulforaphane is a powerful phytochemical (isothiocyanate) that increases enzymes in your liver that help destroy cancer-causing chemicals you may consume or be exposed to in your environment. It is also known to block inflammation and damage to joint cartilage.[18]

Because of the power of these phytochemicals, I highly encourage you to sprout your own broccoli seeds and eat fresh organic broccoli as often as possible. It's hard to beat these two wholesome foods for their phytonutrients and fiber.

However, there may be times when you want far larger amounts of these two incredible compounds. For those times, I recommend taking broccoli sprout powder or broccoli seed extract. I sell a fermented version of broccoli sprout powder on my website, because fermentation helps convert glucoraphanin into sulforaphane before you even ingest it. Again, if you are taking the seeds as mentioned previously, you will not need this supplement as it is in the seeds naturally.

BINDERS

If you don't consume binders when you're fasting, you run the risk of resorbing the toxins you so carefully were able to remove from your fat, thus exposing yourself to more damage from the toxins you've unleashed from the safe cocoons of your fat cells. A binder does just what it sounds like it should do: it binds with substances in the GI tract so that those substances can be excreted through the feces.

There are a large number of binders on the market and one can make an argument for using many of them. I recommend using all of the ones below based on my review of the literature[19] and personal experience. All binders need to be taken on an empty stomach, either one hour before or two hours after your KetoFast meal. If you take the binders too close to when you eat food, the binders will actually bind the nutrients found in the food and make them unavailable, rendering them essentially useless.

Activated charcoal: 5 to 6 grams. Activated charcoal is the primary filtration mechanism for most home water filter systems because it is so effective at removing chlorine, disinfection by-products, and drugs that are in the water supply. It has been used to remove lead[20] and to treat iron overdose[21] and mercury poisoning.[22] Taken at the appropriate time (not too close to when you eat your KetoFast meal), it will help eliminate the toxins that the liver is releasing into the bile and subsequently into the colon via your stool.

Chitosan: 2 to 3 grams. Chitosan is a derivative of chitin, which is a naturally fibrous material found in the exoskeletons of crustaceans and insects.[23] It has been shown to be useful in removing heavy metals[24, 25, 26] and even radionuclides.[27]

Modified citrus pectin: 5 grams. Pectin, a complex carbohydrate found in virtually all plants, helps bind cells together and maintain the shape and integrity of cell membranes. A modified form of citrus pectin derived from the pulp and peel of citrus fruits has been shown to attach to cancer cells to prevent them from spreading throughout the body, pointing the way to a potentially safe approach for preventing or reducing cancer metastases.[28] It is also very effective for binding heavy metals.[29, 30]

Chlorella: 4 to 10 grams. Chlorophyll has a number of important biological activities, several of which offer protection against cancer. These include:[31, 32]

- Binding to carcinogenic chemicals—such as polycyclic aromatic hydrocarbons from tobacco smoke, heterocyclic amines from cooked meat, and aflatoxin-B1 (a mycotoxin found in moldy peanuts and other grains and legumes)—and allowing your body to safely eliminate them

- Antioxidant effects, decreasing cellular damage caused by carcinogenic chemicals and radiation

- Inhibiting cytochrome P450 enzymes, which are required for the activation of pro-carcinogens, thus helping decrease your risk of chemically induced cancers

Dark green vegetables are a rich source of chlorophyll. Another excellent source, indeed one of the best, is chlorella, a green alga often recommended as a binder in heavy metal detoxification protocols. Chlorella has a particular affinity for binding and eliminating mercury, and can therefore be useful when eating a lot of fish. It's also high in plant-based protein.

I typically take 10 grams, or 50 of the fermented chlorella tablets that I sell on my website, mercola.com, before my last meal or before I walk in the sunshine, as there is some evidence that it increases adenosine triphosphate (ATP) production in the mitochondria.[33] Chlorella is one of the most chlorophyll-dense foods, and 10 grams of chlorella is equivalent to the chlorophyll in several pounds of spinach. One of the most important factors to consider when purchasing a chlorella product is its digestibility. The key to its detoxing abilities lies *within* the membrane of this single cell, but the cell wall of chlorella is actually indigestible to humans.

Broken cell wall is the term most often used to describe chlorella that has been rendered digestible. If a product does not specify that the cell wall has been broken, you're likely flushing your money down the toilet, as the chlorella will simply pass right through you without doing you any good.

SUPPORTING YOUR KETOFAST
WITH SAUNA THERAPY

One of the primary ways that your body excretes toxins is through your sweat, so doing things that encourage sweating is an important part of KetoFasting. As you'll soon learn, not all forms of sweating are effective at releasing toxins. The good news is that you won't need to exert yourself to work up a cleansing sweat. In fact, the ideal way to excrete toxins through your sweat is to relax in a specific type of sauna. But before I get into the specifics of sauna bathing, let's take a look at what toxins might be lurking in your sweat.

Some of the toxins that researchers have found lurking in sweat include phthalates (a chemical family found in everyday consumer products);[1] cadmium and mercury, and bisphenol A (BPA).

BPA is a ubiquitous chemical contaminant found in the lining of cans, on-the-go drink bottles, shower curtains, and receipts, to name just a few everyday items you may be exposed to. It was identified in the sweat of 80 percent of the participants in one 2012 study, even in some individuals who had no BPA detected in serum, blood, or urine.[2]

Cadmium is a carcinogenic heavy metal that is typically used in batteries and pigments, but has also been found in jewelry sold in large chain stores as recently as 2018.[3] Notably, cadmium has been found to be concentrated in sweat more than in blood plasma, and mercury levels have been found to normalize with repeated sauna use.[4]

Another study evaluated the blood, urine, and sweat from 20 individuals and analyzed them for approximately 120 compounds.[5] According to the authors: "Many toxic elements appear to be preferentially excreted through sweat. Presumably stored in tissues, some toxic elements readily identified in the perspiration of some participants were not found in their serum. Induced sweating appears to be a potential method for elimination of many toxic elements from the human body."

HOW TO INCREASE DETOXIFICATION THROUGH YOUR SWEAT

While it is certainly possible to do KetoFasting without access to a sauna, it is not ideal, and you will not experience as many of the benefits. Remember, one of the primary benefits of KetoFasting is to help you eliminate toxins, and it is very difficult to do this optimally without access to a sauna. The best type to use is a near-infrared sauna. If at all possible, it should be in your home so it is convenient and you will use it. Cost is an issue for many, so I discuss some inexpensive options below.

The Difference between Active and Passive Sweating

While you could exercise to sweat, active sweating is not the same as passive sweating and it will not release as many toxins. Perhaps even more important, when you are KetoFasting you really don't want to engage in vigorous exercise, as this will impair your body's ability to maximize the benefits of partial fasting.

Again, while you certainly can sweat up a storm with exercise, if you're working on detoxifying heavy metals and other pernicious toxins from your body, passive sweating is far more effective than active sweating. Active sweating is caused by physical exertion such as during exercise. Research has shown the toxin concentration in sweat during exercise is actually quite low.

Sweat samples taken during sauna bathing, on the other hand—i.e., during passive sweating—reveal that high amounts of toxins are being released in the sweat. The reason for this has to do with sympathetic versus parasympathetic nervous system activation. Your autonomic nervous system has two states, commonly referred to as "fight or flight" and "rest and digest."

When you're exercising vigorously enough to start sweating, your body is allocating energy toward your muscles, lungs, and heart. There's no cellular reserves or hormonal gearing for detoxification or cellular repair or anything like that. During passive sweating, however, your body is heated, which helps release toxins through your sweat. Since you're not exerting yourself in any way, your body is able to use the energy generated from the incandescent heat lamps to heal and repair itself.

THE DIFFERENCES BETWEEN NEAR- AND FAR-INFRARED SAUNAS

The vast majority of infrared (IR) saunas are far IR. While these certainly have many benefits, they also have many drawbacks. The difference between far and near IR is the wavelength of the light. Many people (including me until relatively recently when I studied this more carefully) don't understand the penetration of the two types of saunas.

Near-infrared light is just beyond the light spectrum of visible red light; it starts around 700 nanometers and goes up to 1,400 nanometers. Mid-infrared ranges from 1,400 to 3,000 nanometers, and far infrared is from 3,000 to 100,000 nanometers.

It is important to understand these frequencies, as they have significant biological consequences. Near IR actually can penetrate into your body up to 100 millimeters (3.9 inches), while far IR only penetrates a few millimeters, or a tiny fraction of an inch. Even though far IR has more energy than near IR, water in your body absorbs the radiation from far IR before it can penetrate effectively into your tissues.

Let me explain. Water absorbs different wavelengths to different degrees. Water actually starts absorbing the energy at about 980 nanometers—right in the middle of the near-IR spectrum. But it's a continuum, so once you get out of near IR, at about 1,400 or 1,500 nanometers, the water is absorbing nearly all the wavelengths and virtually none of infrared is entering your body. Once you get out to mid-IR, and certainly when you get to far-IR wavelengths, they're 100 percent absorbed by water. This means that far-IR saunas are essentially surface-heating you, and heating you in a conductive fashion. With near-IR wavelengths, you get radiant, penetrating heat. This is a much more efficient way to heat biological tissues.

You can observe a similar effect when you are outside on a sunny summer day and feel the heat of the sun on your skin. When a cloud passes over, the warmth instantly disappears. Did you ever wonder why? It's because clouds are loaded with water and they absorb the far-infrared; it never reaches your skin, so you don't heat up.

Near IR Activates Your Body's Innate Capacity for Healing

Most people who have done some level of studying natural health understand how important regular sunlight exposure is to our health. And nearly everyone understands that exposure to sunlight creates vitamin D in your skin (far better than swallowing vitamin D capsules). It is exposure to ultraviolet B (UVB) wavelengths that causes your body to make vitamin D.

Traditionally, the benefit of sun exposure is thought to be almost universally due to UVB radiation. You might be surprised to learn that UVB in sunlight is less than one-half of 1 percent of the sunlight spectrum, while 40 percent of sunlight—yes, 40 percent, or nearly 100 times more than UVB—is in the near-IR spectrum. This strongly supports the idea that near IR is an important frequency to be exposed to.

Photobiomodulation (PBM) is the term used to describe light's beneficial effects in your body. Interestingly, near IR has a number of wavelengths that can activate proteins called cytochromes in your mitochondria's electron transport chain. This activation helps your mitochondria become more efficient in producing energy.

Far-IR frequencies do not appear to have any PBM impacts on your mitochondria. In addition to activating your mitochondria, near IR and red light that is also present in heat lamp bulbs helps to structure the water in your body and provide it with energy that can be used in a variety of different ways.

So now you understand that sunlight exposure is doing more than heating your body or promoting vitamin D production. It actually activates an entirely different healing system. Since you have mitochondria in every cell of your body, with the exception of red blood cells, it's a core restorative healing system.

Far-IR Saunas Often Misrepresent Their Benefits

There's a great deal of confusion on this issue, and many sauna makers take advantage of that confusion. Makers of far-IR saunas often promote their products as doing exactly what near-IR saunas do. But remember, far-IR saunas are NOT providing radiant heat; they heat your body by conduction, which is why you have to heat them up to a relatively high temperature before you go in or you simply won't sweat.

Beware of "Full-Spectrum" Far-IR Sauna Claims

Two other common problems with far-IR saunas are that a) they claim to be "full-spectrum," when in fact they emit virtually no near IR; and b) they emit high levels of electromagnetic fields (EMFs), even while claiming to be low- or no-EMF-emitting.

I've measured many of these low-EMF far-IR saunas, and while there were many with very low *magnetic* fields (the "M" in EMF), they virtually all emitted high amounts of *electric* fields (the "E" in EMF) and many had extraordinarily high and dangerous electric fields.

There are many so-called full-spectrum far-IR saunas available now that have far-IR emitters for heat, but they've added in near-IR emitters in one of two ways. One way is to use LEDs. You can make digital LEDs now that emit only a few monochromatic near-IR wavelengths and not the full range of more than 700

frequencies in the near-IR spectrum. But it still doesn't have the same natural spectral power curve shape as an incandescent bulb, or as the sunlight.

There are also some saunas that use low-energy near-IR emitters that are basically heating elements that are hotter than the far IRs. They do emit a small amount of near IR, but it's at a very low power level, what is termed *irradiance* in light therapy, which has very little biological impact.

The Benefits of Incandescent Near-IR Heating

The incandescent light bulb is the most efficient way to heat tissue because it is almost exclusively full-spectrum near IR. While incandescent light bulbs use far more energy than LED bulbs, the heating they provide has profound therapeutic benefits. Farmers have long used incandescent light bulbs to incubate animal life and keep livestock warm, for example. Incandescent light bulbs can also be used for incandescent sauna therapy.

Sadly, the U.S. and most of Europe have shifted to LEDs and fluorescents to reduce energy consumption. Doing so has removed many of the healing wavelengths of light for the sake of energy efficiency, but with very detrimental consequences to your health. It's not just about detox. It's the vasodilation, the blood circulation, and the structuring of water. There are so many aspects that are beneficial to us.

While it can be quite difficult to find incandescent light bulbs these days, and they cost more than LEDs, you can still find the 250-watt incandescent heat lamps for sauna therapy. You just need to make sure they have no Teflon coating, as the Teflon will vaporize fluoride into your sauna, which is not a great health strategy.

Therapeutic Dosing

Even with light therapy, you don't want excessive exposure. Just like you can't be in the sun for an unlimited amount of time, you don't want to be in the sauna for eight hours. With the sauna, you're going to heat-shock your body—raising cell temperature a few degrees to get detox responses. This works out to a 20- to 30-minute near-IR sauna session delivering the appropriate amount of energy (around 36 to 54 joules at 1½ to 2 feet from the bulbs).

Essentially, what you're doing with near-IR sauna therapy is stimulating your mitochondria to release nitric oxide (NO) and boosting ATP production. Together, your mitochondria, NO, and ATP work in concert to promote healing effects, such as DNA repair and cellular regeneration.

Accessing Your Own Incandescent Sauna

There are a number of companies that produce heat lamp near-IR saunas. SaunaSpace is one of the best, as it has a no-EMF version that not only has no electric and magnetic fields, but also shields against radiofrequency waves from cell phones and Wi-Fi and creates an ideal parasympathetic detox environment. However, they are expensive.

The least-expensive approach would be to build your own near-IR sauna with Teflon-free heat lamps. Instructions can be found in Dr. Lawrence Wilson's book *Sauna Therapy for Detoxification and Healing*, available on Amazon. This type of sauna was used in Dr. John Harvey Kellogg's sanitariums and spas in the early 1900s.

The core of the sauna is made up of four 250-watt Philips incandescent bulbs, which can be purchased for less than $40. You just want to make sure the bulbs you buy do not have a Teflon coating (which some bulbs do, to prevent breakage). When heated, the Teflon emits harmful chemicals. Avoid Teflon to ensure you're not vaporizing fluoride and breathing it in.

Although far less expensive, this approach does present some challenges. First are the materials, as they need to be toxin free and hypoallergenic, which means they can be harder to find and tend to cost more than their more readily available counterparts. Natural materials are best and off-gassing plastics should be avoided.

Second, the bulbs get very hot. You don't want to touch the surface of an incandescent bulb, which can burn. To protect yourself, you need something professionally designed. A hardware cloth or some flexible wire is typically not sufficient.

The third alternative and midtier cost would be a hybrid approach. You can purchase the fixtures and bulb protectors from companies that sell near-IR saunas and use your own enclosure. The fixtures are typically diamond-shaped with one bulb on the top and bottom and two bulbs in the middle.

The heating you want occurs as a result of the light shining onto your body, so you don't really need a sauna tent. But you do need the air around you to be above body temperature, preferably above 100 degrees Fahrenheit, which happens very quickly once you turn the bulbs on. You can hang the heat-lamp-bulb fixture in your shower or even a dedicated closet or small room. Just be careful when using a small room; if surrounding materials like paint or finished wood or carpet have petrochemicals in them, undesirable toxic off-gassing can occur. Also, since the heating is directional, remember to rotate your body so that different parts are exposed.

If you already have a far-IR wood sauna, you could use the near-IR bulb fixture in there—not by turning the sauna on, but by using its four walls, ceiling, and floor as your enclosure.

HOW TO USE A SAUNA SAFELY

Moderate use of a sauna is safe for most people. However, if you have a heart condition, it is wise to consult with your physician first. Further precautions include:

- **Take care to collect or wash away the toxins you sweat out.** Whatever system you use, you will need to use towels to collect your sweat, unless you are in a shower where you can rinse them down the drain. It is also wise to do a cold shower immediately after your sauna, as this will help remove the toxins you are sweating out.

- **Choose a low- or no-EMF near-infrared sauna.** If you are going to use an infrared sauna regularly, be sure it's one that emits low or no nonnative electromagnetic fields (EMFs). This is important, because in addition to causing cellular disturbances throughout the body, EMFs also activate your sympathetic nervous system, which will hamper your detox efforts.

  If you are purchasing a sauna, make sure the manufacturer supplies you with third-party analysis that shows its levels of near infrared (in the 800 to 850 nanometer range) are just as high as the far infrared. Most saunas have far-infrared levels that are 20 times higher than near infrared. It's important to do your homework before making such an important health investment.

- **Stay safe.** Avoid using a sauna alone, as a sudden drop in blood pressure or dehydration may lead to a potentially lethal situation. Avoid the sauna if you are pregnant or if you are ill. Return to the sauna only after you are feeling better, don't have a fever, and are fully hydrated.

  Always listen to your body when deciding how much heat stress you can tolerate. If you've never used a sauna, you may need to start with just four minutes the first time, adding 30 seconds to each subsequent sauna until you reach 15 to 30 minutes. In some cases, the detoxification process may be severe. This schedule helps your body to slowly acclimate to sweating and eliminating toxins.

- **Avoid alcohol.** Alcohol in combination with sauna therapy increases your risk of arrhythmia, hypotension (extremely low blood pressure), dehydration, and sudden death. In a study from Finland, researchers found that those who experienced sudden death within 24 hours of using a sauna had a high probability of consuming alcohol at the time.[6]

  Avoid the sauna if you've had too much to drink in the past 24 hours as well. While you may have heard sauna use will shorten a hangover, it actually increases your risk of dehydration at a time when you are already dehydrated from the alcohol.

- **Prevent dehydration and mineral loss.** Sauna use increases the amount of fluid you lose through sweating. It's important to replace that fluid by ensuring you are well-hydrated with clean, pure water before using the sauna and paying close attention to rehydrating afterward.

AND NOW FOR THE RECIPES...

I hope that you will enjoy these recipes; Pete and I put a lot of care into creating them. (I hope you'll also enjoy the beautiful photos that were taken in Pete's own kitchen!) I think you'll find the soups, snacks, and teas on the pages that follow are so tasty and nourishing that you'll want to eat them on your non-fasting days too.

As you embark on KetoFasting, I want to congratulate you on taking your wellness into your own hands. Here's to your continued efforts to take control of your health.

PART II

RECIPES

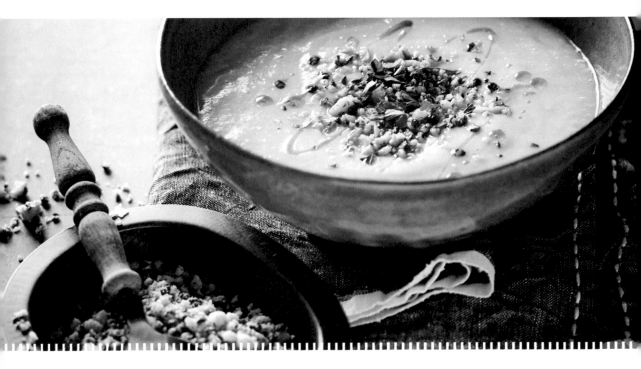

SOUPS

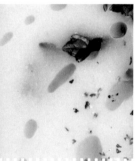
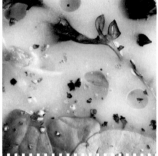
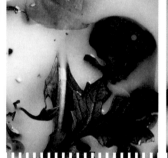
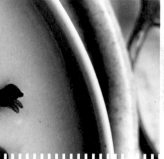

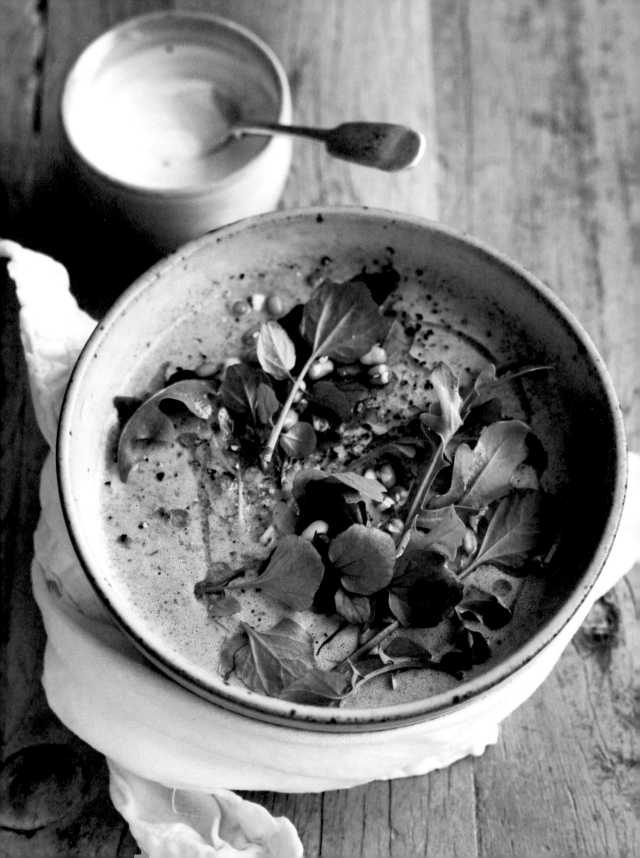

ARUGULA SOUP WITH SPROUTED MUNG BEANS

Using arugula gives this soup a lovely pepperiness and light bitterness that Pete encourages everyone to eat more of to accustom our palates to these wonderful flavors. If you're looking to give up sugar, Pete's advice is to train your taste buds to appreciate more bitter, astringent, and sour foods. Pete firmly believes that there is a world waiting to be discovered if we are open to experimenting with different ingredients. When you travel, you see how different cultures around the world use these ingredients as part of their staple diet, such as bitter melon (bitter gourd) in Asian cultures, bitter endive in European cultures, and astringent foods—such as pomegranate, turmeric, and lentils—in Indian culture. Give this arugula soup a go during your fast. When the fast is over, you can add in a poached egg or even some wild-caught salmon to turn it into a satisfying meal.

Melt the fat in a small saucepan over medium heat. Add the onion and garlic and cook for 3 minutes, or until softened. Stir in the spinach, broth, and half the arugula and bring to a boil. Cover, reduce the heat to low, and gently simmer for 15 minutes.

Blend the soup with a handheld blender until almost smooth. Season with salt and pepper to taste. Add some lemon juice just to taste.

Ladle the soup into a warm bowl, then add the watercress and the remaining arugula.

Top with mung beans, coconut yogurt, and olive oil and serve.

Serves: 1

1 Tbsp coconut oil or good-quality animal fat

¼ small onion, chopped

1 garlic clove, finely chopped

¼ cup baby spinach leaves

1¾ cups Chicken Bone Broth (page 164; you can substitute beef broth or pork broth)

⅓ cup baby arugula, divided

Sea salt and freshly ground black pepper

Lemon juice, to taste

2 Tbsp watercress

2 Tbsp sprouted mung beans

½ Tbsp coconut yogurt, to serve

Extra-virgin olive oil, to serve

NUTRITION INFORMATION

calories 292.1 | 25.2g total fat (15.1g saturated fat, 0.1g trans fat) | 4.6mg cholesterol
611.2mg sodium | 6.4g total carbohydrate (0.9g dietary fiber, 2.2g total sugars, -g added sugars)
10.9g protein | 0.1mcg vitamin D | 53.4mg calcium | 1.4mg iron | 505.3mg potassium

ASIAN TURNIP AND CABBAGE SOUP

The combination of Asian aromatics in a broth is a delicious and quick meal. This is Pete's go-to dish as he always has a supply of fresh ginger and spring onions. Pete likes to use these two ingredients with a lot of his dishes as they can enliven humble scrambled eggs and serve as an excellent spice for steamed wild fish or even grass-fed organic beef. Here Pete has used ginger and spring onions to add some vibrancy to a simple broth and added vegetables.

Serves: 1

1 Tbsp coconut oil or good-quality animal fat

1 Tbsp julienned ginger

1¾ cups Beef Bone Broth (page 163; you can substitute chicken broth or pork broth)

1 tsp tamari

¼ tsp finely grated fresh turmeric or ground turmeric

½ cup diced turnips, cut into ½-inch dice

¼ cup shredded Chinese cabbage

1 Tbsp finely sliced spring onions

1 tsp fish sauce, plus more to taste

1 tsp lemon juice, plus more to taste

Heat the oil or fat in a small saucepan over medium heat. Add the ginger and cook for 30 seconds, until fragrant.

Add the broth, tamari, and turmeric and bring to a boil, then reduce the heat to low. Add the turnips, cover with a lid, and gently simmer for 15 minutes.

Add the cabbage and onions and simmer for 3 minutes, or until wilted.

Add the fish sauce and lemon juice.

Ladle the soup into a warm bowl and serve.

NUTRITION INFORMATION

calories 236.3 | 18.1g total fat (12.6g saturated fat, 0.1g trans fat) | 3.9mg cholesterol 1362.5mg sodium | 8.9g total carbohydrate (1.8g dietary fiber, 4g total sugars, -g added sugars) 10g protein | 0.1mcg vitamin D | 60.3mg calcium | 1.7mg iron | 565.5mg potassium

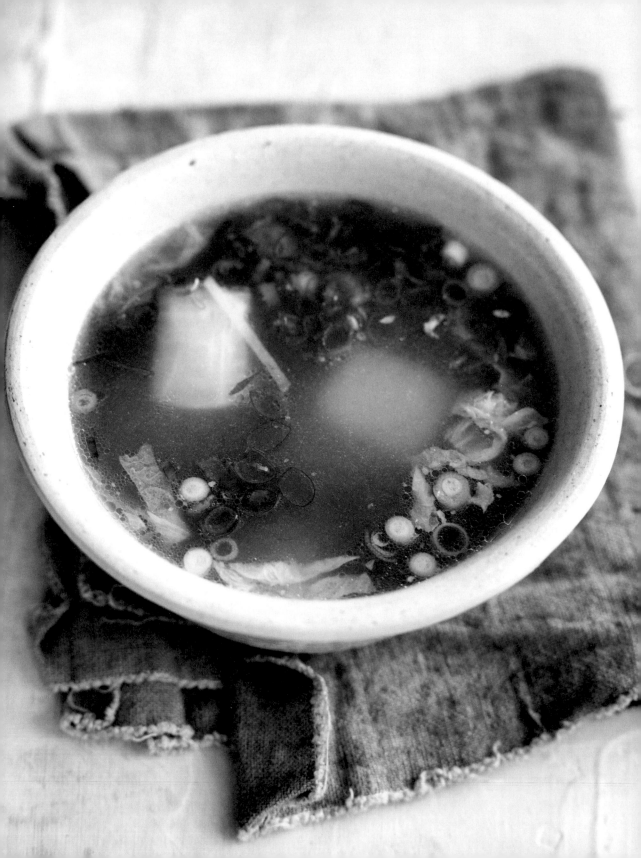

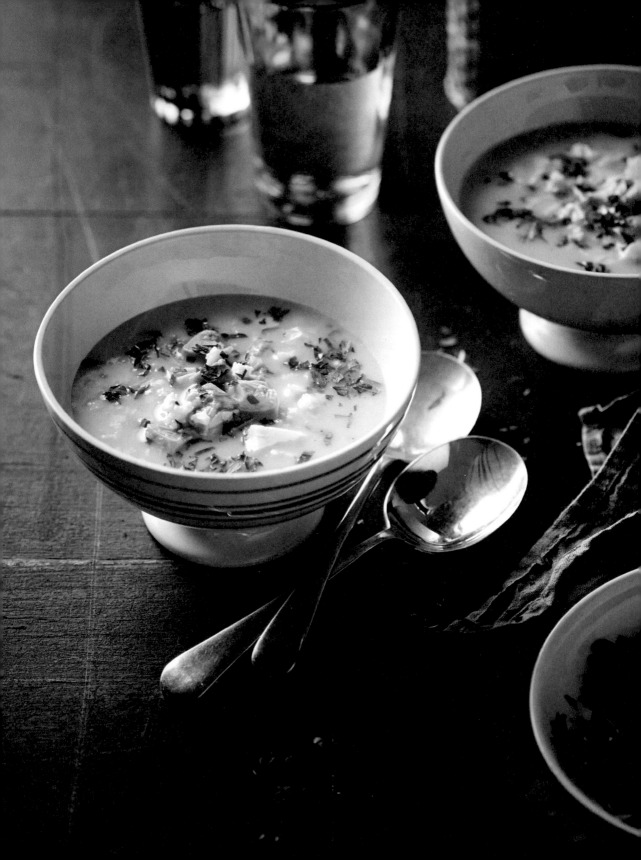

AVGOLEMONO SOUP

This soup contains all of Pete's favorite components: yummy chicken bone broth, eggs, lemon, herbs, and chicken. This classic Greek dish is a winner in the cooler months and can be on the table in a short period of time. If you like, you can add extra vegetables such as broccoli or zucchini rice, parsnip noodles, silverbeet, or asparagus.

Place the cauliflower in the bowl of a food processor and pulse into tiny, fine pieces that look like rice. Set aside.

Heat the oil or fat in a saucepan over medium heat. Add the onion and sauté until soft and translucent, about 5 to 6 minutes. Add the garlic and sauté for 1 minute, or until fragrant.

Pour in the broth and bring to a boil, then reduce the heat to low.

Add the diced chicken and cauliflower rice to the broth and simmer, stirring occasionally, for 10 minutes, or until the chicken is cooked through.

Crack the eggs into a large bowl and whisk in the lemon juice. Slowly pour in 2 cups of the hot chicken broth in a steady stream, whisking constantly, until combined. Then, whisking the chicken broth vigorously, slowly incorporate the warm lemon and egg mixture into the soup until creamy and cloudy looking.

Season to taste with salt, pepper, and more lemon juice. Serve immediately with the parsley sprinkled on top.

Serves: 4

½ head of cauliflower (about 1⅓ pounds)

4 Tbsp coconut oil

2 small onions, finely chopped

1 garlic clove, finely chopped

6 cups Chicken Bone Broth (page 164)

2 chicken thigh fillets, diced small

3 eggs

4 Tbsp lemon juice, plus extra to taste

Sea salt and freshly ground black pepper

2 Tbsp chopped flat-leaf parsley, to serve

NUTRITION INFORMATION

calories 351.6 | 25.8g total fat (15g saturated fat, 0.1g trans fat) | 183.6mg cholesterol
730.5mg sodium | 13.5g total carbohydrate (3g dietary fiber, 4.9g total sugars, 0g added sugars)
19.7g protein | 0.1mcg vitamin D | 73.3mg calcium | 2.4mg iron | 745mg potassium

BOK CHOY AND GINGER SOUP

In this soup Pete paired bok choy with ginger, which is a very medicinal ingredient. These two ingredients blend so well together that many dishes feature the combination, including this basic broth. It will no doubt become one of your favorite soups to enjoy not only during your fast, but well into the future. To add a little more substance to the broth when you are not on the fast, try it with some wild salmon that has been lightly poached, with 100 percent grass-fed organic sausages, or even with a couple of poached eggs for something different. Whichever way you go, just have fun.

Serves: 1

1 Tbsp coconut oil or good-quality animal fat

1 garlic clove, finely chopped

2 Tbsp julienned ginger

1½ cups Chicken Bone Broth (page 164; you can substitute beef, pork, or fish broth)

1½ tsp tamari

½ tsp sesame oil

½ head baby bok choy, trimmed, roughly chopped

½ spring onion, chopped

⅛ cup sprouted mung beans

½ tsp sliced long red chili (optional)

Sea salt and freshly ground black pepper

Heat the oil or fat in a small saucepan over medium heat. Add the garlic and ginger and cook for 1 minute, or until soft.

Add the broth, tamari, and sesame oil to the saucepan, stir, and bring to a simmer over medium heat. Turn down the heat to low and gently simmer for 20 minutes.

Add the bok choy, onions, mung beans, and chili (if using) and continue to simmer for 5 minutes, or until the vegetables are tender. Season with salt and pepper to taste.

Ladle the broth into a warm bowl and serve.

NUTRITION INFORMATION

calories 306.4 | 21.4g total fat (13.1g saturated fat, 0.1g trans fat) | 4.2mg cholesterol
1471.6mg sodium | 15.7g total carbohydrate (5.1g dietary fiber, 6.7g total sugars, -g added sugars
16.8g protein | 0.1mcg vitamin D | 477mg calcium | 4.8mg iron | 1516.4mg potassium

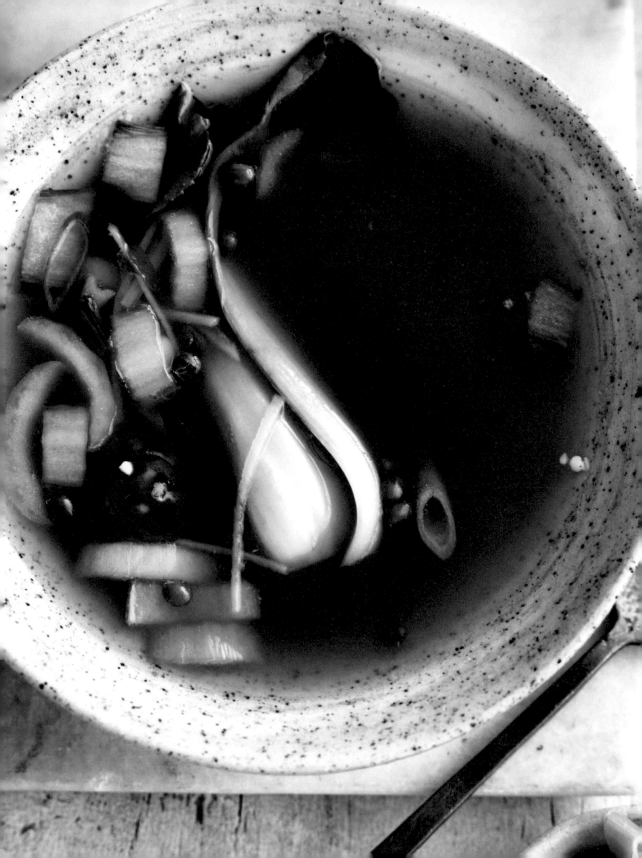

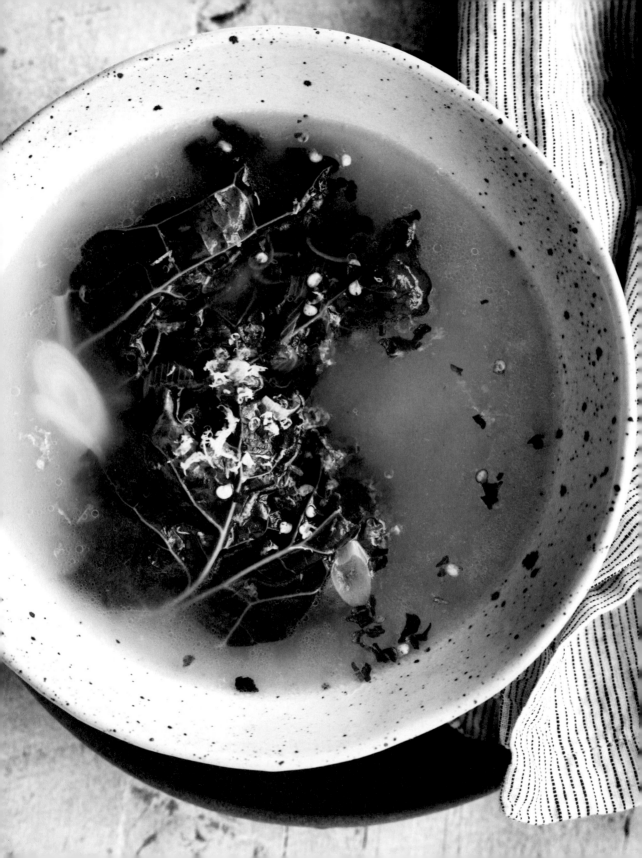

BRAISED KALE SOUP

Pete's philosophy is very simple when it comes to cooking and that is: make it super tasty, make it easy, and make it with the best possible ingredients that have been grown, raised, farmed, or caught with integrity. If you follow these rules you really cannot go wrong. Take this recipe, for example. Admittedly, it is for our fasting book, so it is very easy, but you could quite easily turn this soup into a meal for the family by adding some organic grass-fed and grass-finished meatballs or poaching some wild salmon into it. Always have broth in the freezer for these times and a delicious, healthy meal will only be minutes away.

Heat the oil or fat in a saucepan over medium heat. Add the onion and garlic and cook for 3 minutes, or until soft. Pour in the broth, bring to a boil, then simmer over low heat for 15 minutes.

Add the kale and continue to simmer for 5 minutes, or until wilted. Season with salt and pepper to taste.

Ladle the broth into a bowl and top with chili flakes, if desired.

Serves: 1

1 Tbsp coconut oil or good-quality animal fat

¼ small onion, thinly sliced

1 garlic clove, finely chopped

1¾ cups Chicken Bone Broth (page 164)

¼ cup torn kale, leafy part only

Sea salt and freshly ground black pepper

Pinch of chili flakes (optional)

NUTRITION INFORMATION

calories 226.7 | 18.3g total fat (12.6g saturated fat, 0.1g trans fat) | 3.9mg cholesterol
668.8mg sodium | 6.8g total carbohydrate (1.2g dietary fiber, 2.2g total sugars, -g added sugars)
9.4g protein | 0.1mcg vitamin D | 62mg calcium | 1.5mg iron | 468.4mg potassium

CABBAGE AND BRUSSELS SPROUT SOUP

Cabbage soup is a versatile and highly nutritious staple. In this recipe Pete wanted to show how delicious a cabbage soup can be and added in turmeric, which is a wonderful medicinal ingredient that not only benefits our bodies, but also adds delicious flavor. The addition of brussels sprouts provides some depth. When you are not doing your fast, you can add some protein such as wild prawns, organic chicken, or any other well-sourced animal protein that you enjoy.

Serves: 1

1 Tbsp coconut oil or good-quality animal fat

¼ small onion, chopped

1 garlic clove, finely chopped

½ cup shredded green cabbage

2 ounces (about 4) brussels sprouts, halved

1¾ cups Chicken Bone Broth (page 164; you can substitute beef broth or pork broth)

1 bay leaf

¼ tsp freshly grated turmeric or ground turmeric

Sea salt and freshly ground black pepper

Heat the oil or fat in a saucepan over medium heat. Add the onion and garlic and cook for 5 minutes, or until the onion is translucent.

Add the cabbage, brussels sprouts, broth, bay leaf, and turmeric and stir well to combine.

Bring to a boil. Reduce the heat to low, cover with a lid, and simmer gently for 20 minutes, or until the vegetables are tender. Season with salt and pepper to taste.

Ladle the soup into a warm bowl and serve.

NUTRITION INFORMATION

calories 256.4 | 18.5g total fat (12.7g saturated fat, 0.1g trans fat) | 4.2mg cholesterol
716.1mg sodium | 12.7g total carbohydrate (3.8g dietary fiber, 4.5g total sugars, -g added sugars)
11.4g protein | 0.1mcg vitamin D | 74.8mg calcium | 2.4mg iron | 681.6mg potassium

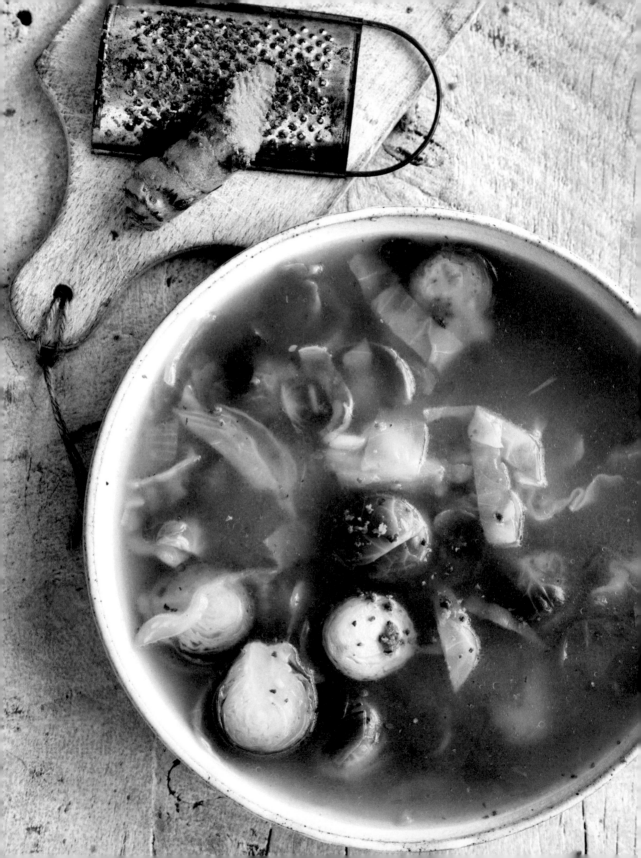

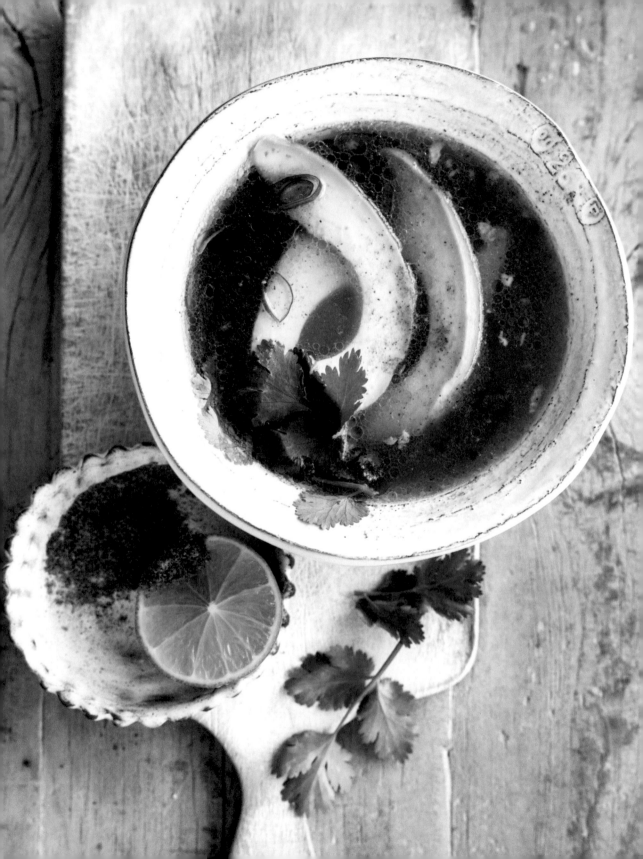

CHICKEN BROTH
WITH AVOCADO

This may seem like the strangest recipe in the book, but trust me and give it a try before you dismiss the idea of having avocado in a warm or hot soup. Pete was fortunate enough to visit Mexico recently on a culinary journey and this was one of the revelations for him on that trip. The lightly spiced Mexican broth that has chicken broth as its base and just-warm slices of avocado is so nourishing. After every bite it became more and more addictive, where each mouthful was better than the last. When not fasting, you may like to add in some chicken, prawns or fish, and/or an egg that is either soft-boiled or raw (just whisk it in at the end of cooking so the soup becomes thicker) to make this a larger meal for breakfast, lunch, or dinner.

Heat the broth in a saucepan until hot and season with a pinch of salt and pepper. Transfer the broth to a bowl, then add the avocado, sprinkle the Mexican spices over, and garnish with the cilantro and onions. Squeeze some lime juice over, if desired, and serve.

Serves: 1

1¾ cups Chicken Bone Broth (page 164)

Sea salt and freshly ground black pepper

½ avocado, sliced

¼ to ½ tsp Mexican spice blend (or more, if desired)

2 sprigs cilantro

1 tsp sliced spring onions, to serve

1 lime wedge, to serve (optional)

NUTRITION INFORMATION

calories 243.6 | 19.7g total fat (3.5g saturated fat, 0.1g trans fat) | 4.2mg cholesterol
701.2mg sodium | 9g total carbohydrate (5g dietary fiber, 1.3g total sugars, 0g added sugars)
10.1g protein | 0.1mcg vitamin D | 37.1mg calcium | 1.5mg iron | 740.1mg potassium

CHILLED AVOCADO SOUP

Pete planted four different varieties of avocado trees on his property and cannot wait for the harvest in coming years. He realizes he's going to have avocados in abundance! He has a chest freezer in preparation for this, so he can blend and store the avocados to last throughout the year.

This recipe can be whipped up in a matter of minutes and is a wonderful source of good fats. To make it a more substantial meal, just add some cooked crabmeat, prawns, chicken, or bacon.

Serves: 4

2 cups Chicken Bone Broth (page 164), plus extra if needed

1½ cups coconut milk

1½ tsp grated ginger

½ tsp ground cumin

2 avocados, pitted and peeled

1 large handful cilantro, chopped

1 Tbsp lime juice

Sea salt and freshly ground black pepper

1 handful watercress

Pumpkin seeds (activated if possible, i.e., soaked for 4 to 8 hours in salted water), to serve

1 diced Lebanese cucumber, to serve

Place the broth, coconut milk, ginger, and cumin in a large saucepan and bring to a boil over medium heat. Reduce the heat to medium-low and simmer for 5 minutes.

Remove from the heat and leave to cool.

Once cool, pour the soup into a blender. Add the avocado flesh, cilantro, and lime juice and blend until smooth and creamy. Add more broth or water to thin if necessary. Season to taste with salt and pepper. Place in the fridge to chill, or serve at room temperature, if desired.

Ladle the soup into bowls, sprinkle some watercress over, and scatter the pumpkin seeds and diced cucumber on top.

NUTRITION INFORMATION

calories 194.6 | 15.9g total fat (4g saturated fat, 0g trans fat) | 1.3mg cholesterol
186.2mg sodium | 10.7g total carbohydrate (5.9g dietary fiber, 1.9g total sugars, -g added sugars)
6.1g protein | 1.4mcg vitamin D | 87.4mg calcium | 1.7mg iron | 669.9mg potassium

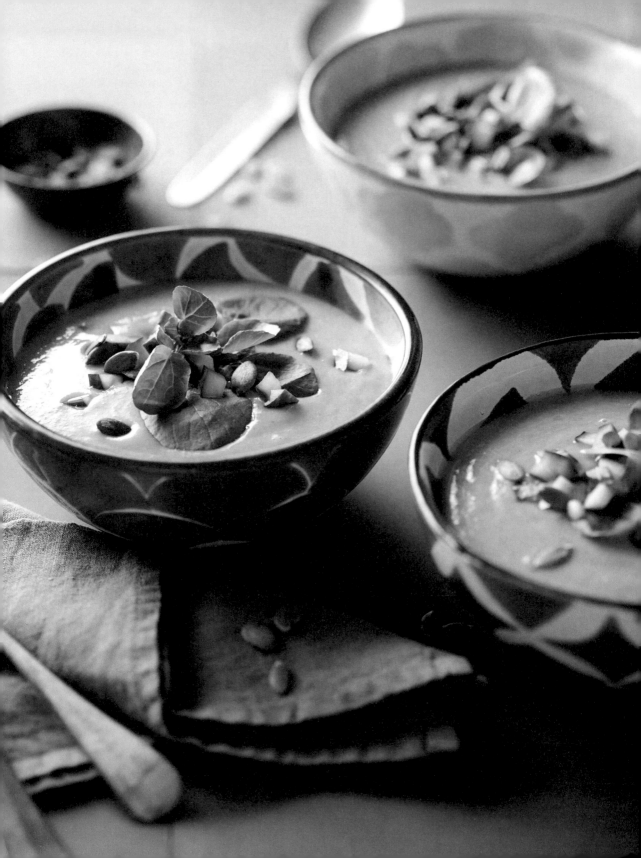

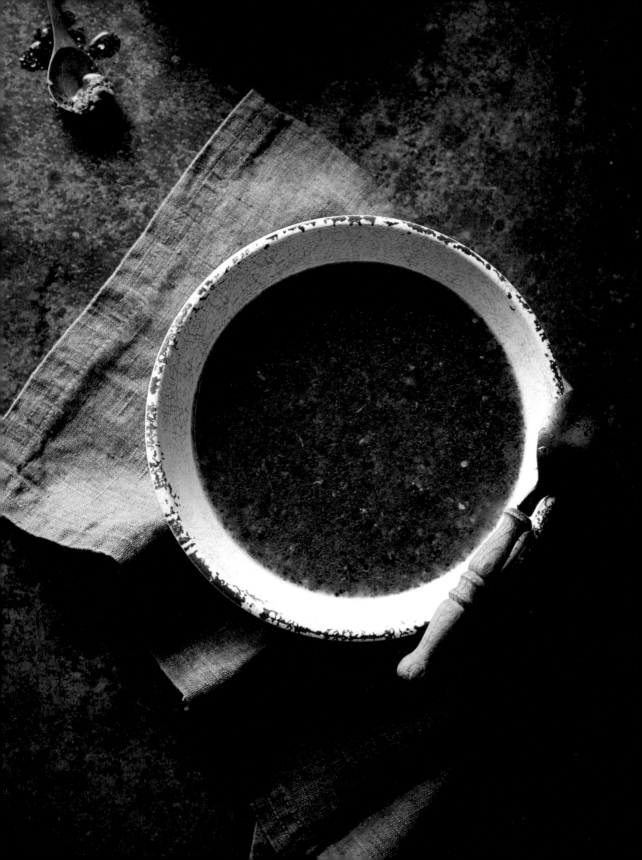

CHIMICHURRI BONE BROTH

Bone broth is well known for its health-giving properties, and we encourage everyone to incorporate it into their diet. This age-old recipe is dirt cheap—about 20 to 30 cents per serving—and sustainable, using all parts of the animal, which are good things in anyone's book. If you're having your daily broth, then you might like to jazz it up a little from time to time with different spices or herbs. Here is something to do when you have leftover chimichurri. Adding the chimichurri to the broth takes it to another level, and as a bonus you get all those wonderful herbs into your system, too.

Pour the broth into a saucepan and bring to a simmer. Remove from the heat and stir in ½ cup of chimichurri. Season to taste with salt and pepper.

Ladle the broth into soup bowls or mugs and serve.

Serves: 4

4 cups Chicken Bone Broth, Beef Bone Broth, or Fish Broth (pages 164, 163, and 167)

Chimichurri (see recipe below)

Sea salt and freshly ground black pepper

CHIMICHURRI

To make the chimichurri, place the garlic and a little salt in a mortar and crush with the pestle. Add the jalapeño, parsley, and cilantro and pound to a paste. Stir in the vinegar, cumin, and olive oil. Season to taste with pepper and more salt. If you prefer, you could also make the chimichurri in a food processor.

Makes: ¾ cup

3 garlic cloves, peeled

Sea salt

1 jalapeño or long red chili, seeded and finely chopped

1 very large handful flat-leaf parsley leaves

1 very large handful cilantro

3 Tbsp apple cider vinegar

1 tsp ground cumin

3 Tbsp olive oil or melted coconut oil

Freshly ground black pepper

NUTRITION INFORMATION

calories 123.8 | 9.9g total fat (1.8g saturated fat, 0g trans fat) | 2.6mg cholesterol
495mg sodium | 3.2g total carbohydrate (0.6g dietary fiber, 1.1g total sugars, 0g added sugars)
6g protein | 0.1mcg vitamin D | 31.6mg calcium | 1.5mg iron | 314.4mg potassium

CHINESE CABBAGE
AND MUNG BEAN SOUP

Every single Chinese restaurant has a list of soups to choose from that all come from their base ingredient, which is always an aromatic broth of some sort. Chicken broth, seafood broth, pork broth, duck broth, and other types of broths that are made from the simple art of simmering animal bones with water and aromatic ingredients are the foundation for these amazing soups. Here Pete used chicken broth and added some Chinese cabbage along with mung bean sprouts for texture and little crunchy toasted sesame seeds for good measure.

Serves: 1

1 Tbsp coconut oil or good-quality animal fat

¼ onion, chopped

½ tsp finely grated ginger

1 garlic clove, finely chopped

½ tsp finely chopped coriander root

1¾ cups Chicken Bone Broth (page 164) (you can substitute pork, beef, or fish broth)

1½ Tbsp sprouted mung beans

½ tsp tamari or coconut aminos

1 tsp fish sauce

¼ tsp sesame oil

⅛ tsp ground turmeric

⅓ cup shredded Chinese cabbage

½ spring onion (green part only), julienned

¼ tsp toasted sesame seeds

1 tsp chopped cilantro

Heat the oil or fat in a small saucepan over medium heat. Add the onion and cook for 3 minutes, or until translucent. Add the ginger, garlic, and coriander root and cook for 30 seconds, or until fragrant.

Add the broth and bring to a boil. Turn down the heat to medium-low, then add the mung beans, tamari, fish sauce, sesame oil, and turmeric and simmer for 15 minutes, or until the vegetables are tender.

Stir in the cabbage and spring onions and cook for 3 minutes, or until the cabbage is wilted. Add a little salt and pepper to taste, if desired.

Ladle the soup into a warm bowl. Sprinkle the toasted sesame seeds and chopped cilantro on top and serve.

NUTRITION INFORMATION

calories 257 | 19.9g total fat (12.9g saturated fat, 0.1g trans fat) | 4.2mg cholesterol
1339.7mg sodium | 9.3g total carbohydrate (2g dietary fiber, 3.5g total sugars, -g added sugars)
11.3g protein | 0.1mcg vitamin D | 77.9mg calcium | 1.9mg iron | 589.7mg potassium

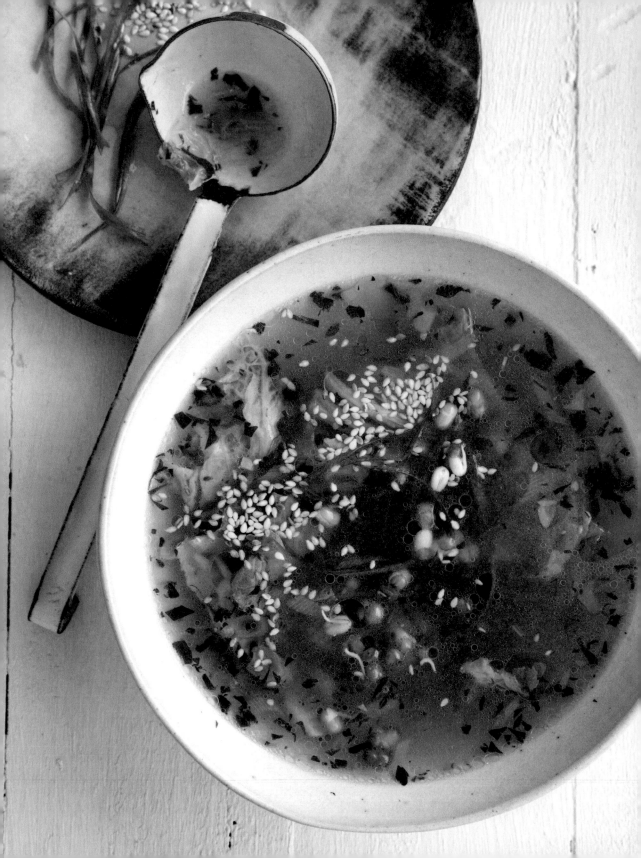

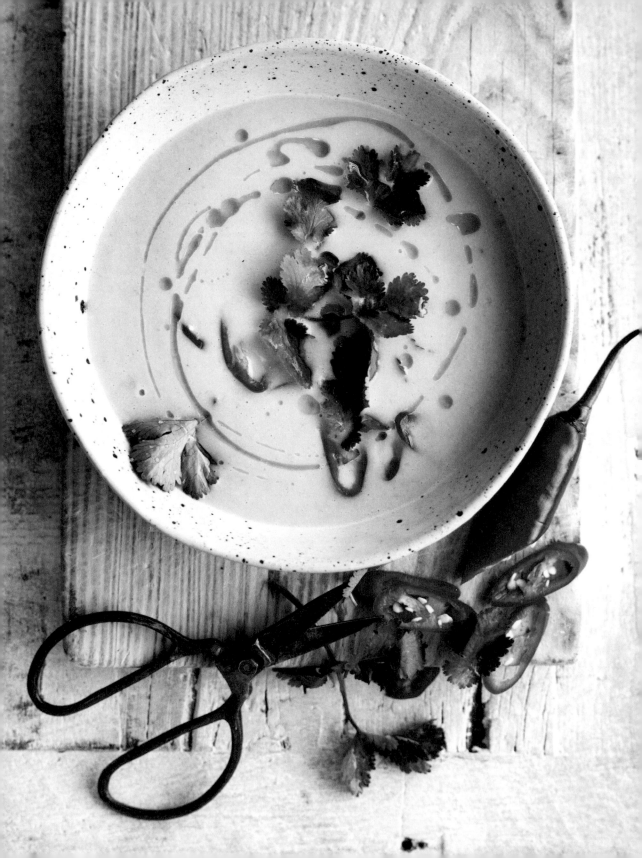

CREAMY CURRIED CAULIFLOWER SOUP

Pete is a lover of creamy soups as they bring him back to his childhood and those memories of a comforting bowl of delicious goodness in the winter months. He wanted to re-create those feelings with a mouthwatering soup that is anti-inflammatory and has all the ingredients that nourish our body and soul.

In this soup, cauliflower and broth are equal stars with gentle spices added to tantalize the taste buds and bring a smile to your face. It's ideal to make a big batch and freeze the leftovers for when the weather is cold and you feel like a quick bowl of goodness.

Melt the oil or fat in a small saucepan over medium heat. Add the onion and cook for 3 minutes, or until softened. Add the garlic, ginger, and spices and cook for 30 seconds, or until fragrant. Stir in the cauliflower and broth and bring to a boil. Cover with a lid, reduce the heat to low, and simmer for 20 minutes, or until the cauliflower is tender.

Add the coconut cream and lemon juice, then blend the soup with a handheld blender until smooth. Season with salt and pepper to taste.

Ladle the soup into a warm bowl, drizzle some olive oil on top, and finish with sliced chili (if using) and cilantro.

Serves: 1

1 Tbsp coconut oil or good-quality animal fat

¼ small onion, chopped

1 garlic clove, chopped

½ tsp finely chopped ginger

½ tsp ground coriander

½ tsp ground turmeric

1 tsp ground cumin

Small pinch chili powder or cayenne pepper (optional)

1 cup cauliflower, chopped

1¾ cups Chicken Bone Broth (page 164; you can substitute beef broth or pork broth)

2 Tbsp coconut cream

½ tsp lemon juice

Sea salt and freshly ground black pepper

1 tsp extra-virgin olive oil, to serve

¼ long chili, thinly sliced (optional)

3 cilantro sprigs

NUTRITION INFORMATION

calories 369.5 | 31.1g total fat (20.3g saturated fat, 0.1g trans fat) | 4.2mg cholesterol
731.4mg sodium | 11.2g total carbohydrate (2.8g dietary fiber, 3.9g total sugars, -g added sugars)
11.8g protein | 0.1mcg vitamin D | 70.9mg calcium | 3.6mg iron | 780.7mg potassium

CREAMY TURNIP SOUP
WITH MESCLUN

Many people think that turnips are related to the potato family, but in fact they are in the cruciferous family that contains vegetables such as cabbage, broccoli, and cauliflower. Turnips are low in carbs and full of beneficial nutrients that our bodies love. The wonderful thing about using turnips in your cooking is that when they are in season and abundant, they are relatively cheap and can be used in so many different preparations—from raw in salads, to fermented in krauts and kimchi where they add a wonderful flavor and texture, to pickled, and also cooked in soups and roasts. Here Pete lightly spiced the soup and added some fresh lettuce leaves for texture.

Serves: 1

1 Tbsp coconut oil or good-quality animal fat

¼ small onion, chopped

1 garlic clove, finely chopped

½ medium (3 ounces) turnip, ¼-inch diced

¼ cup chopped cauliflower

¼ tsp finely chopped rosemary

1¾ cups Chicken Bone Broth (page 164; you can substitute beef broth or pork broth)

⅛ tsp ground nutmeg

Sea salt and freshly ground black pepper

⅛ cup baby salad green leaves, to garnish

½ tsp olive oil, to serve

Heat the oil or fat in a saucepan over medium heat. Add the onion and cook for 3 minutes, or until translucent.

Add the garlic and cook for 30 seconds, or until fragrant.

Add the turnip, cauliflower, rosemary, and broth and bring to a boil. Reduce the heat to low and gently simmer for 20 minutes, or until the vegetables are tender.

Blend the soup to a smooth consistency using a handheld blender. Stir in the nutmeg and season with salt and pepper to taste.

Ladle the soup into a warm bowl. Scatter a few baby salad green leaves on top, drizzle with olive oil, and finish with a grind of black pepper.

NUTRITION INFORMATION

calories 268.8 | 20.8g total fat (13.1g saturated fat, 0.1g trans fat) | 4.2mg cholesterol
756mg sodium | 10.9g total carbohydrate (2.5g dietary fiber, 5g total sugars, -g added sugars)
10.2g protein | 0.1mcg vitamin D | 67mg calcium | 1.5mg iron | 619mg potassium

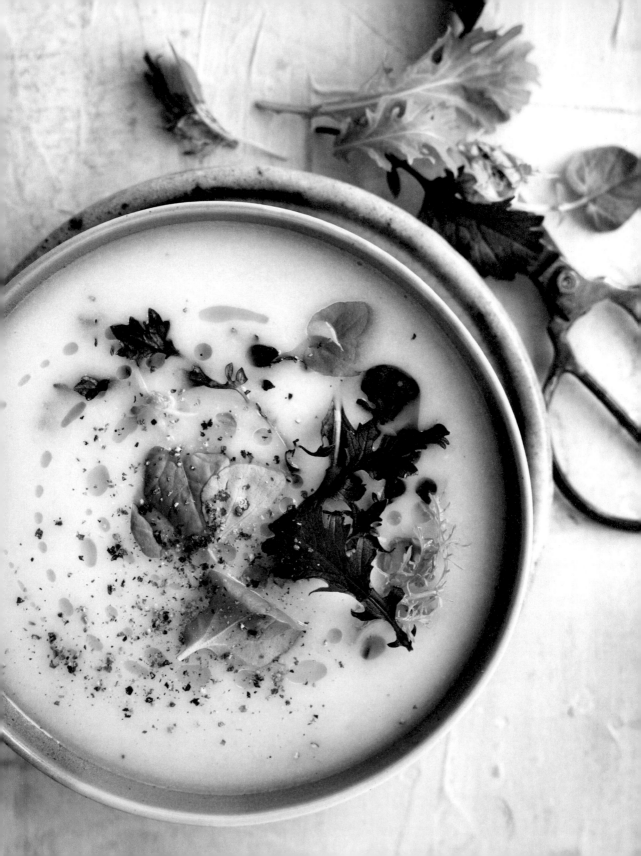

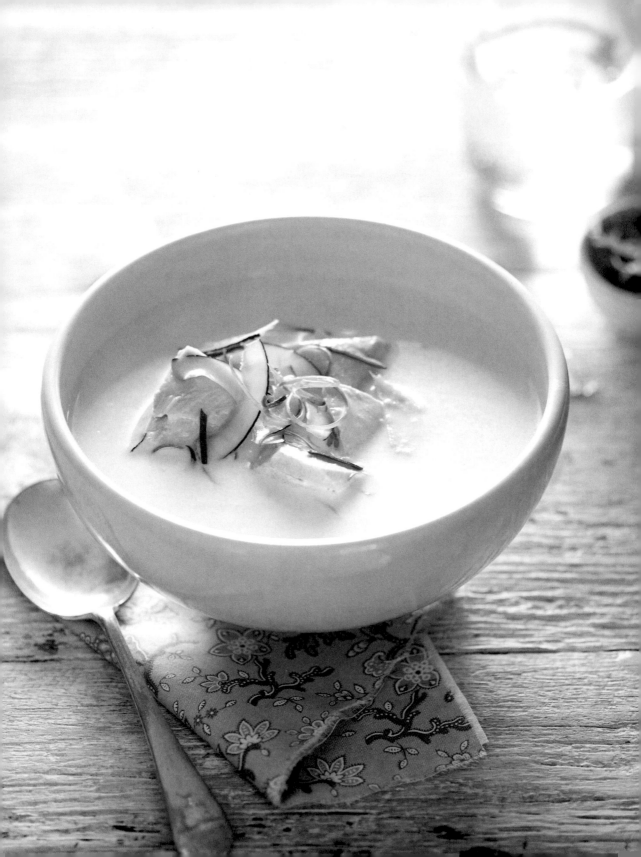

FIJIAN FISH SOUP

Every year Pete spends a week or two in Fiji, where he likes to work alongside the locals and share recipes. One of Pete's favorites is this soup. It is simple yet it delivers so many flavors and is a great way to use up the frames and heads of fish so that nothing goes to waste.

Place the fish heads and carcasses in a large saucepan with 2 quarts of filtered water. Add the salt, onion, peppercorns, and chili and bring to a simmer. Simmer for about 20 minutes, skimming periodically.

Strain the stock into another large saucepan and season to taste with salt and pepper. Stir in the lemon juice, coconut cream, and fish and reheat over low heat for 4 to 5 minutes, or until the fish is cooked through. Be careful not to let the soup boil, as the coconut cream might separate and the fish might overcook.

Ladle the soup into bowls and garnish with spring onions, chili, and coconut shavings.

Serves: 4 to 6

2 lb fish heads and carcasses, such as cod or snapper

2 tsp sea salt

1 large onion, sliced

1 tsp black peppercorns, lightly crushed

1 small red chili, roughly chopped

Sea salt and freshly ground black pepper

1 Tbsp lemon juice

2½ cups coconut cream

½ lb fish fillets (such as snapper, cod, or barramundi), cut into 1-inch cubes

Finely sliced spring onions, to serve

Finely sliced red chili, to serve

Toasted coconut shavings, to serve

NUTRITION INFORMATION

calories 422.9 | 33.5g total fat (28.1g saturated fat, 0g trans fat) | 22.6mg cholesterol
1473.7mg sodium | 7.4g total carbohydrate (1g dietary fiber, 4g total sugars, -g added sugars)
21.9g protein | 0mcg vitamin D | 121.1mg calcium | 0.9mg iron | 826.8mg potassium

FRENCH ONION SOUP

How can anyone say no to a French onion soup that is full of delicious, gut-healing beef broth, health-giving onion (known for regulating blood sugar), and medicinal garlic and thyme? Enjoy this when you want a nourishing breakfast, lunch, or dinner. If you are looking for a heartier dish, add some bone marrow, braised short ribs, or beef cheek.

Serves: 4 to 6

2 Tbsp coconut oil or good-quality animal fat

1¼ lb onions, sliced

3 garlic cloves, chopped

2 tsp finely chopped thyme leaves

6 cups Beef or Chicken Bone Broth (pages 163 and 164) or Vegetable Broth (page 172)

2 bay leaves

Sea salt and freshly ground black pepper

2 macadamia nuts (activated if possible, i.e., soaked for 4 to 8 hours in salted water), finely grated, to serve

A few slices of Paleo or keto bread, to serve (optional)

Heat the oil or fat in a large, heavy-based saucepan over medium-high heat. Add the onion and cook, stirring occasionally, for 30 minutes or until the onion is soft and beginning to brown.

Add the garlic and thyme; reduce the heat to medium-low and cook, stirring occasionally, for 30 minutes, or until the onion is caramelized.

Increase the heat to medium and, stirring constantly, gradually pour in the broth, then add the bay leaves.

Bring to a boil, skimming off any scum that rises to the surface. Reduce the heat to low and simmer gently for 50 minutes, until the soup is full of flavor with a nicely balanced sweetness. Season to taste with salt and pepper.

Ladle the soup into bowls, sprinkle some grated macadamia over the top, and serve with some Paleo bread on the side.

NUTRITION INFORMATION

calories 177.2 | 12.7g total fat (8.5g saturated fat, 0g trans fat) | 2.6mg cholesterol
345.3mg sodium | 9.8g total carbohydrate (1.5g dietary fiber, 4g total sugars, -g added sugars)
6.4g protein | 0.1mcg vitamin D | 39.3mg calcium | 1mg iron | 341.3mg potassium

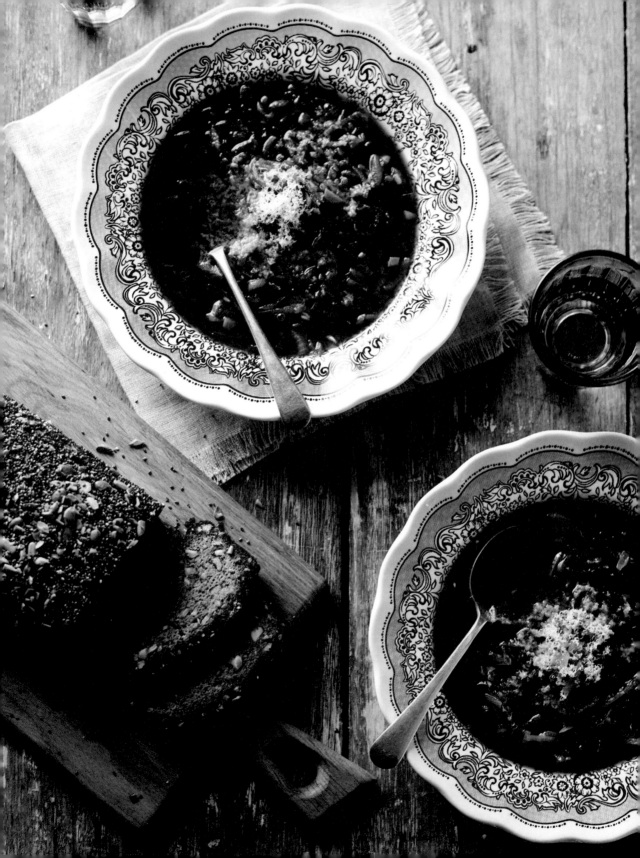

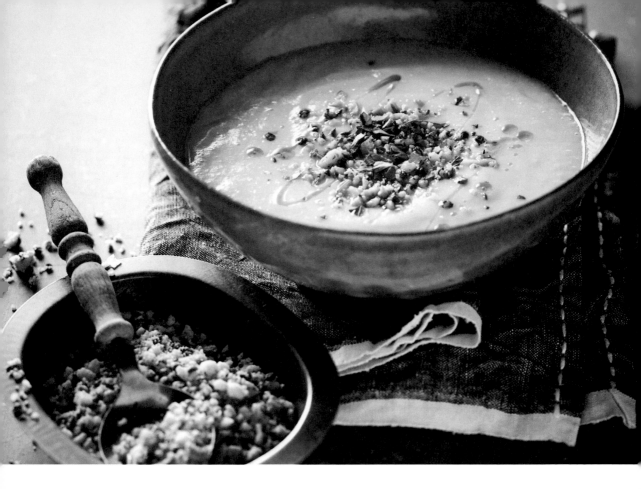

TURMERIC OIL

Makes: ½ cup

½ cup coconut oil, macadamia oil, or good-quality animal fat

1 tsp ground turmeric

Heat the oil or fat in a saucepan over low heat. Mix in the turmeric and gently simmer for 10 minutes (do not bring to a boil).

Set aside and allow to cool completely before using. Store the turmeric oil in an airtight container and melt before using. If using animal fat, you will need to store your turmeric oil in the fridge.

HEALING GARLIC SOUP

Pete can't count the number of times he has been asked, "What is great to eat when you have a cold or flu?" Apart from drinking water with some lemon juice in it, Pete thoroughly recommends this warming and nourishing soup, which is chock-full of goodness: garlic, onion, leek, chicken broth, and good-quality fats.

Melt the coconut oil in a large saucepan over medium heat. Add the garlic, onion, and leek and sauté, stirring occasionally, for 5 minutes, or until the vegetables are softened and fragrant.

Pour in the broth, add the parsnip, and simmer for 30 minutes, or until the vegetables are tender.

Puree the soup with a handheld blender. Add the nutmeg and season to taste with salt and pepper. Reheat the soup over low heat.

Place the egg yolks and olive oil in a bowl and whisk to combine. Add a ladle of the hot soup to the egg mixture and whisk to incorporate. Pour the warm egg mixture into the soup and stir gently for 1 minute to heat through. Do not allow the soup to boil or the egg yolks will curdle.

Ladle the soup into warm bowls. Sprinkle the almonds and parsley on top and drizzle with a little turmeric oil.

Serves: 4 to 6

3 Tbsp coconut oil or good-quality animal fat

32 garlic cloves, roughly chopped

1 onion, chopped

1 leek (white part only), rinsed well and chopped

6 cups Chicken Bone Broth (page 164)

1 parsnip, chopped

2 pinches freshly grated nutmeg

Sea salt and freshly ground black pepper

4 egg yolks

3 Tbsp olive oil

¼ lb almonds (activated if possible, i.e., soaked for 4 to 8 hours in salted water), toasted and chopped

2 Tbsp chopped flat-leaf parsley leaves

Drizzle of Turmeric Oil (page 86)

NUTRITION INFORMATION
calories 485.3 | 38.7g total fat (13.5g saturated fat, 0.1g trans fat) | 184.1mg cholesterol
531.7mg sodium | 20.4g total carbohydrate (4g dietary fiber, 3.8g total sugars, -g added sugars)
16.8g protein | 1mcg vitamin D | 154.4mg calcium | 3mg iron | 668.8mg potassium

INDIAN-SPICED CAULIFLOWER SOUP

Mustard seeds and curry leaves popping in the bottom of a saucepan creates a delightfully seductive aroma. This soup is a wonderful example of how carefully blended spices can enhance a humble vegetable. If you have never roasted cauliflower before, then Pete urges you to try, as he believes this is the best technique for showing off the beautiful flavor of this vegetable. Play around with different spice combinations, or for the best snack just sprinkle on some cumin and sea salt and roast until golden. The key is to roast the cauliflower until it is nearly burned—not black, but a beautiful, deep golden brown.

Serves: 4

4 Tbsp coconut oil, divided

1 cauliflower head, cut into florets (see tip)

1 garlic clove, finely chopped

Garam Masala (page 89)

Sea salt

1 Tbsp yellow mustard seeds

10 curry leaves

2 onions, chopped

1 pinch cayenne pepper

3 cups Chicken Bone Broth or Vegetable Broth (pages 164 and 172)

1½ tsp apple cider vinegar

Freshly ground black pepper

1 small handful cilantro, to serve

Toasted cumin seeds, to serve

Preheat the oven to 390°F.

Melt 2 tablespoons of the coconut oil. Toss the cauliflower florets and garlic with the melted coconut oil and about ⅓ of the garam masala on a large baking sheet. Sprinkle on a little salt and roast for about 25 minutes, or until the cauliflower is golden and the garlic is aromatic.

Remove from the oven and set aside.

Heat the remaining coconut oil in a large saucepan over medium-high heat. Add the mustard seeds and curry leaves and cook for 1 minute. Add the onion and cook for 3 to 4 minutes, or until softened.

Add 1 tablespoon of the garam masala, the cayenne pepper, cauliflower, and garlic and cook for a few minutes, until fragrant. Add the broth and 3 cups of filtered water and bring to a boil. Reduce the heat to low and simmer for 10 to 15 minutes, or until the cauliflower is soft.

Remove from the heat and blend until smooth. Stir in the vinegar. Season to taste with salt and pepper.

Ladle the soup into bowls and top with cilantro, a sprinkle of toasted cumin seeds, and the reserved cauliflower florets, if desired (see tip).

NUTRITION INFORMATION

calories 230.2 | 17.2g total fat (12.3g saturated fat, 0g trans fat) | 2.3mg cholesterol
345.4mg sodium | 12.6g total carbohydrate (3.9g dietary fiber, 4.8g total sugars, 0g added sugars)
8.4g protein | 0.1mcg vitamin D | 60.8mg calcium | 1.5mg iron | 698.1mg potassium

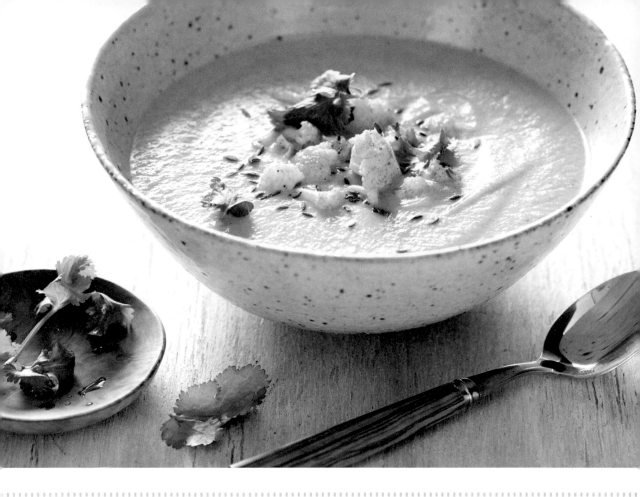

GARAM MASALA

To make the garam masala, toast the spices and seeds in a small saucepan over medium heat, shaking the pan to move them around, for about 3 minutes, or until dark and fragrant. Set aside to cool.

Grind the spices to a fine powder in a spice grinder or using a mortar and pestle.

Makes: ½ cup

3 Tbsp coriander seeds

3 Tbsp cumin seeds

5 to 6 cinnamon sticks, broken into pieces

1 Tbsp cardamom pods

1 Tbsp whole cloves

1 tsp fennel seeds

TIP: The garam masala can be stored in an airtight glass container for up to 3 months.

Also, if you'd like the soup to be chunky, roast an extra ½ head of cauliflower. Use ⅔ of the cauliflower florets to make the soup and add the remaining roasted cauliflower florets to each bowl before serving.

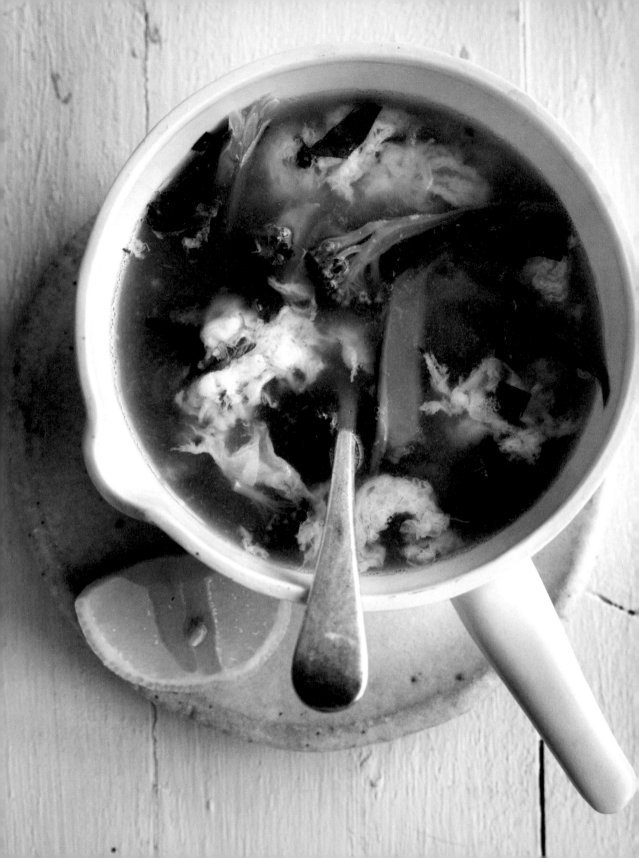

ITALIAN
EGG DROP SOUP

Having read the introduction to this book, you know why it's so essential to make these soups and broths as often as possible. This soup is a traditional family favorite. Add an egg or two for body and delicious flavor, along with a wonderful texture that kids and adults all love. You can add eggs to pretty much any of the soups or broths in this book, if you like.

Pour the broth into a saucepan and bring to a boil, then turn down the heat to a simmer. Add the broccolini and blanch for 5 minutes, or until cooked through. Transfer the broccolini to a chopping board and roughly chop.

Combine the egg and lemon juice in a bowl and beat with a fork. Pour the egg mixture into the broth in the saucepan and stir for 1 minute. Return the broccolini to the pan. Add the parsley, some more lemon juice (if desired), and season with salt and pepper to taste. Spoon the soup into a warm bowl and drizzle some olive oil on top.

Serves: 1

1¾ cups Chicken Bone Broth (page 164)

½ cup broccolini, trimmed

1 egg

1 tsp lemon juice, plus more to taste

1 tsp chopped flat-leaf parsley

Sea salt and freshly ground black pepper

Extra-virgin olive oil, to drizzle

NUTRITION INFORMATION

calories 310.1 | 24.4g total fat (5.1g saturated fat, 0.1g trans fat) | 213.1mg cholesterol
779.8mg sodium | 6.2g total carbohydrate (1.5g dietary fiber, 2.4g total sugars, -g added sugars)
17.1g protein | 1.3mcg vitamin D | 74.9mg calcium | 2.2mg iron | 587.8mg potassium

JAPANESE DAIKON SOUP

Pete believes Japanese cooks are the true masters when it comes to preparing and eating clean food. He feels that they respect the ingredients and let them shine without complicating their beauty. The subtle yet complex flavors of Japanese broths and soups make them sensational. You may wish to use a seaweed broth as the base, though any variety will yield great results.

Serves: 1

1 Tbsp coconut oil or good-quality animal fat

1 garlic clove, finely chopped

1 tsp finely grated ginger

1 tsp chopped spring onions (white part only)

1¾ cups Chicken Bone Broth (page 164; you can substitute beef broth or pork broth)

½ cup daikon, cut into ½-inch cubes

1 tsp sesame oil

1½ tsp tamari or coconut aminos

½ tsp sriracha

5 baby spinach leaves

1 sprig of cilantro

Heat the oil or fat in a small saucepan over medium heat. Add the garlic, ginger, and onions and cook for 30 seconds, until fragrant.

Add the broth and bring to a boil. Turn down the heat to low, then add the daikon, sesame oil, tamari, and sriracha and gently simmer for 20 minutes, or until the daikon is tender.

Add a little salt and pepper to taste, if desired.

Ladle the soup into a warm bowl, stir in the spinach, and garnish with a sprig of cilantro.

NUTRITION INFORMATION

calories 287.2 | 23.1g total fat (13.4g saturated fat, 0.1g trans fat) | 4.2mg cholesterol
1173mg sodium | 9.3g total carbohydrate (2.5g dietary fiber, 3.3g total sugars, -g added sugars)
11.7g protein | 0.1mcg vitamin D | 94.6mg calcium | 2.8mg iron | 831.2mg potassium

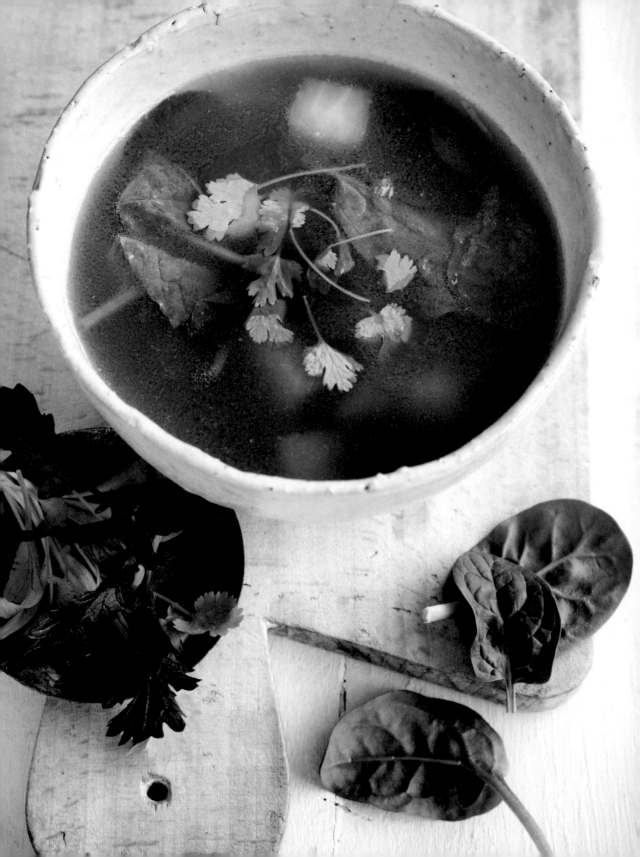

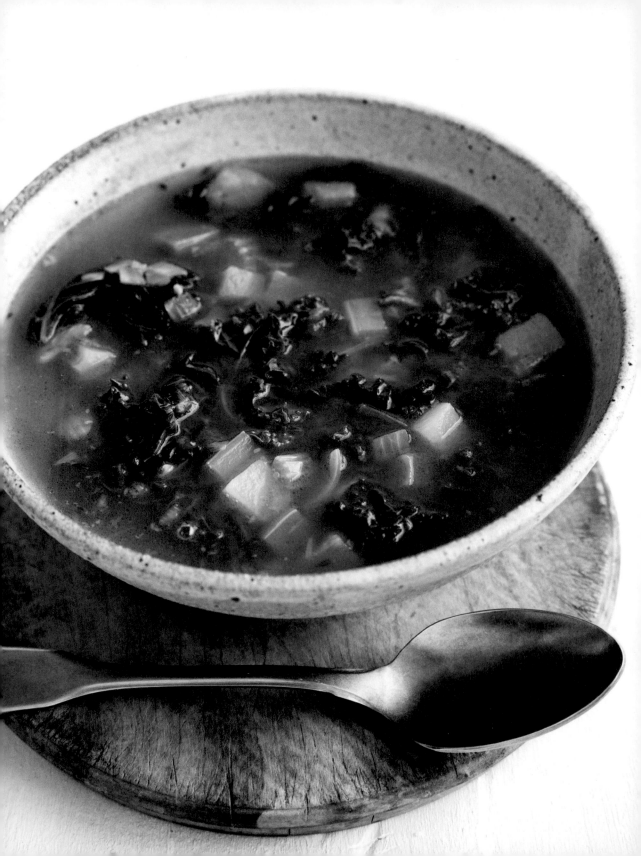

KALE MINESTRONE

One of the most famous soup recipes in the world is the very humble but very "moreish" Italian minestrone (meaning that when you eat it, you want more!). There is no set recipe for minestrone as it is generally made with whatever vegetables are in season and abundant, and the wonderful thing about minestrone is that it is a family favorite. Here we have adapted the recipe to fit in with the formula for fasting and it is still absolutely delicious and satisfying. However, if you want to create a larger meal for when you are not fasting, then adding some meatballs, chicken, or fish into the soup would be delicious, as would a poached egg or two.

Melt the oil or fat in a saucepan over medium heat. Add the onion, garlic, carrot, celery, turnip, and thyme and cook, stirring occasionally, for 5 minutes, or until the vegetables are starting to color. Add the whole peeled tomato, tomato paste, broth, and bay leaf and bring to a boil. Reduce the heat to low, cover, and gently simmer for 20 minutes, or until the vegetables are tender.

Add the kale to the saucepan and continue to cook for 3 minutes, or until wilted. Season with salt and pepper to taste.

Ladle the soup into a warm bowl, sprinkle with parsley, and serve.

Serves: 1

1½ Tbsp coconut oil or good-quality animal fat

¼ small onion, finely sliced

1 garlic clove, finely chopped

½ small carrot, diced

1½ Tbsp diced celery

½ small turnip, diced

½ tsp chopped thyme

¼ cup whole peeled tomatoes, preferably from a jar, crushed

1 tsp tomato paste

1¾ cups Beef or Chicken Bone Broth (pages 163 and 164)

1 bay leaf

⅛ cup roughly chopped kale leaves

Salt and freshly ground black pepper

1 tsp chopped parsley

NUTRITION INFORMATION

calories 337.5 | 25.3g total fat (18.3g saturated fat, 0.1g trans fat) | 4.2mg cholesterol
802.3mg sodium | 17g total carbohydrate (3.5g dietary fiber, 8g total sugars, 0g added sugars)
11.2g protein | 0.1mcg vitamin D | 87.5mg calcium | 1.6mg iron | 771.6mg potassium

KOHLRABI AND CARAMELIZED ONION SOUP WITH MACADAMIA

Kohlrabi has a taste between broccoli and cabbage, so wherever you like to use those ingredients, you can substitute this exciting vegetable. You can use it in cold or cooked dishes, from salads and slaws to soups and sides. Kohlrabi, also called German turnip, is a biennial vegetable—a low, stout cultivar of wild cabbage. It is the same species as cabbage, broccoli, cauliflower, kale, brussels sprout, and collard greens and it can be eaten raw or cooked. Edible preparations are made with both the stem and the leaves, so don't waste any of this precious vegetable. Pete has created a lovely creamy soup with the addition of some macadamia. The flavors work very well together.

Serves: 1

1 Tbsp coconut oil or good-quality animal fat

¼ onion, sliced

¾ cups chopped kohlrabi

1 garlic clove, chopped

1¾ cups Beef Bone Broth (page 163; you can substitute chicken broth or pork broth)

1 bay leaf

Sea salt and freshly ground black pepper

1 macadamia nut, grated

5 watercress sprigs

Heat the oil or fat in a small saucepan over medium-low heat. Add the onion and sauté, stirring frequently, for 8 minutes, or until caramelized. Stir in the kohlrabi and garlic and cook for 30 seconds, or until fragrant.

Pour in the broth, add the bay leaf, and bring to a boil. Turn down the heat to low and gently simmer for 20 minutes, until the kohlrabi is tender. Remove and discard the bay leaf.

Blend the soup to a smooth consistency using a handheld blender. Season with salt and pepper to taste.

To serve, ladle the soup into a warm bowl, sprinkle with the grated macadamia, and garnish with sprigs of watercress.

NUTRITION INFORMATION
calories 267.8 | 20.5g total fat (13g saturated fat, 0.1g trans fat) | 4.2mg cholesterol
714.5mg sodium | 11.9g total carbohydrate (4.3g dietary fiber, 3.7g total sugars, -g added sugars)
11g protein | 0.1mcg vitamin D | 88.7mg calcium | 2.6mg iron | 714.6mg potassium

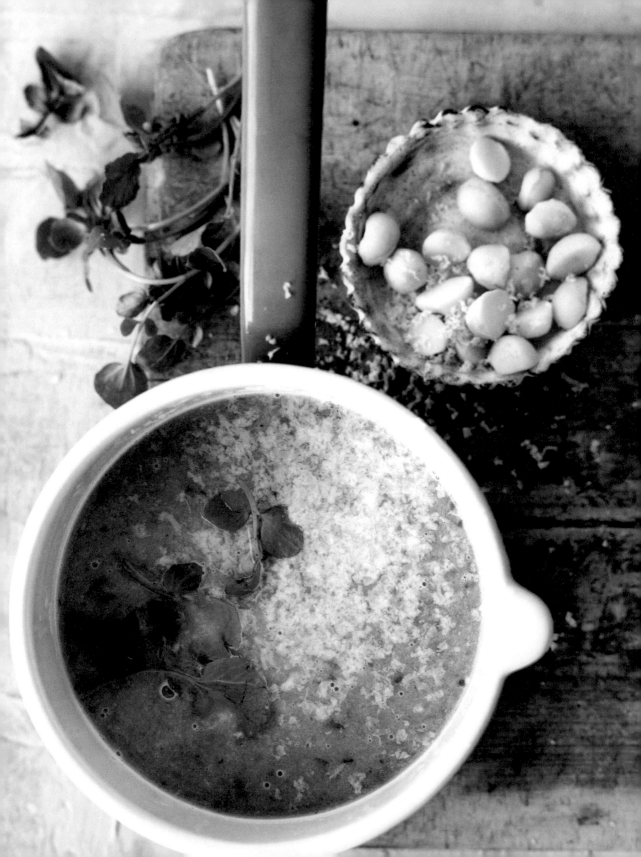

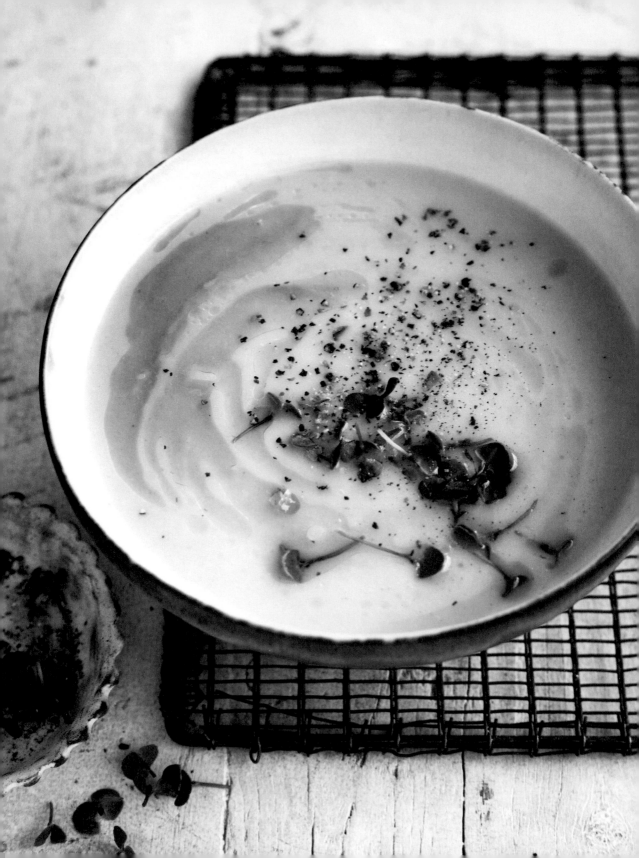

KOHLRABI AND LEEK SOUP

This exquisite soup has become a favorite of Pete's. It contains the freshest ingredients and is served with a splash of olive oil for an added high-quality fat. This soup is truly mouthwatering and will leave you wanting more.

Heat the oil or fat in a saucepan over medium heat. Add the onion and cook for 3 minutes, or until translucent.

Add the leeks, garlic, and kohlrabi and cook for 2 minutes.

Pour in the broth, add the bay leaf, and bring to a boil.

Once the soup starts to boil, reduce the heat to low and simmer for 20 minutes, or until the vegetables are tender. Remove and discard the bay leaf.

Blend the soup to a smooth consistency using a handheld blender. Stir in the nutmeg and season with salt and pepper to taste.

Ladle the soup into a warm bowl, add micro herbs (if using), drizzle with olive oil, and finish with a grind of black pepper.

Serves: 1

1 Tbsp coconut oil or good-quality animal fat

¼ small onion, chopped

⅓ cup leeks (white part only), chopped

1 garlic clove, chopped

½ cup chopped kohlrabi

1¾ cups Chicken Bone Broth (page 164; you can substitute beef broth or pork broth)

1 bay leaf

⅛ tsp nutmeg

Sea salt and freshly ground black pepper

Micro herbs of your choice, to serve (optional)

1 tsp olive oil, to serve

NUTRITION INFORMATION

calories 308.2 | 23.1g total fat (13.4g saturated fat, 0.1g trans fat) | 4.2mg cholesterol
715mg sodium | 15.8g total carbohydrate (3.7g dietary fiber, 5g total sugars, -g added sugars)
10.8g protein | 0.1mcg vitamin D | 81mg calcium | 2.7mg iron | 675.8mg potassium

LAKSA SOUP

Pete's first visit to Malaysia many years ago introduced him to one of their national treasures and most famous delicacies, the ever delicious laksa, which not only seduces you with its tantalizing aromas, but also with the depth of flavor that every spoonful holds. Pete has simplified the recipe to make it easy and quick for you to re-create at home but still keep the essence of the dish in all its beauty. As a bonus, this laksa uses nourishing broth, creamy coconut, and also the medicinal qualities of turmeric as a triple whammy. When not fasting, you can turn this into a larger meal by adding wild-caught shrimp or salmon, organic chicken, or grass-fed beef and mushrooms.

Serves: 1

1 Tbsp coconut oil or good-quality animal fat

1½ Tbsp Paleo Laksa Spice Paste (page 101)

¼ tsp ground turmeric

½ tsp finely grated ginger

½ tsp chopped coriander root and stem

6¾ oz coconut milk

6¾ oz Fish Broth (page 167; you can substitute chicken broth)

¼ cup roughly chopped bok choy

2 tsp fish sauce, or more to taste

½ tsp lime juice, or more to taste

1½ Tbsp finely shredded Chinese cabbage

¼ cup sprouted mung beans

2 to 3 Thai basil leaves

2 to 3 cilantro

Place the oil or fat in a large saucepan over medium heat. Add the spice paste, turmeric, ginger, and coriander and sauté for 1½ minutes, or until fragrant.

Add the coconut milk and broth and bring to a boil. Decrease the heat and simmer for 20 minutes for the flavors to develop.

Add the bok choy and cook for 3 minutes, or until just cooked through.

Stir in the fish sauce, lime juice, cabbage, and mung beans and cook for 1 minute.

Ladle the soup into a warm serving bowl and top with Thai basil and cilantro.

NUTRITION INFORMATION

calories 557.6 | 52.2g total fat (42.9g saturated fat, 0g trans fat) | 2.2mg cholesterol 1819.7mg sodium | 18.4g total carbohydrate (2.9g dietary fiber, 10.9g total sugars, 1.5g added sugars) 10.4g protein | 0.1mcg vitamin D | 85.9mg calcium | 3.1mg iron | 823.7mg potassium

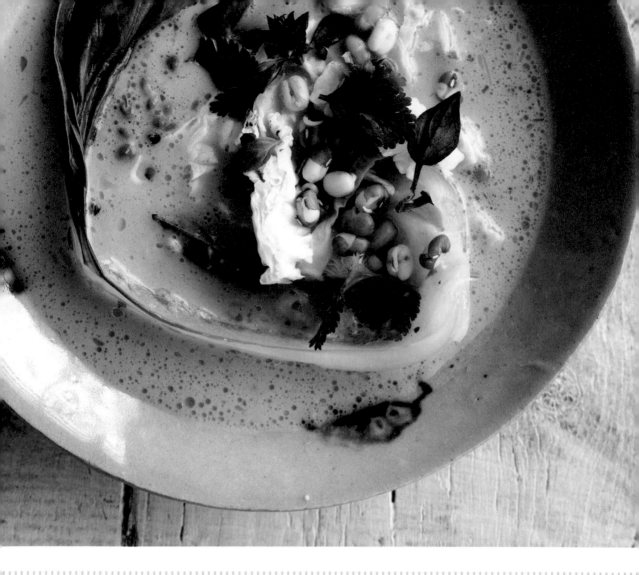

PALEO LAKSA SPICE PASTE

Process the garlic, chilies, lemongrass, turmeric, and lime leaves with 3 tablespoons of water in a high-speed blender or pound using a mortar and pestle until smooth.

Makes: ½ cup

3 garlic cloves, peeled

2 long red chilies (about 3 ounces), seeded and roughly chopped

1 lemongrass stem, white part only, thinly sliced

½ tsp ground turmeric

3 kaffir lime leaves, finely shredded

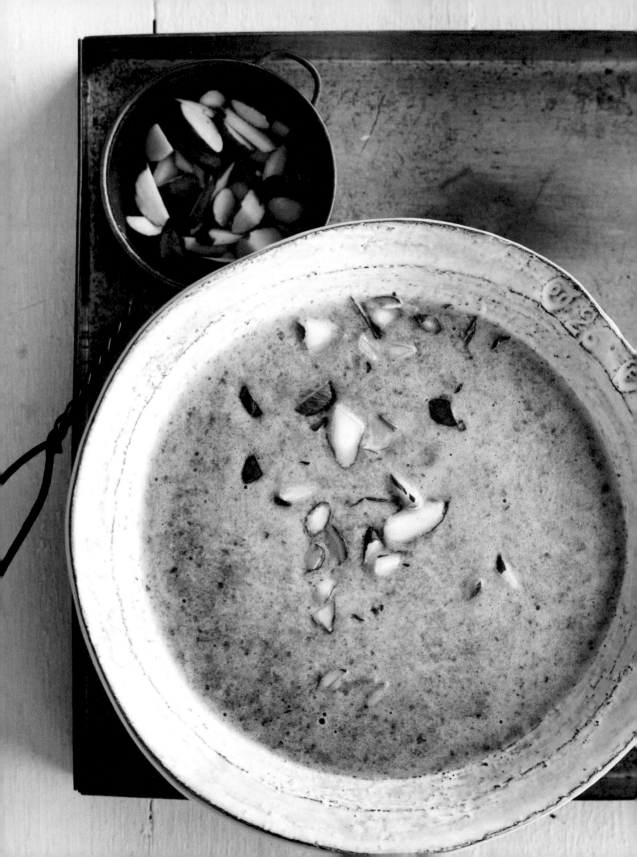

MUSTARD GREENS SOUP
WITH ALMONDS

Mustard greens are becoming more and more popular and are, conveniently, readily available. They are super easy to grow and harvest, and they make for a very versatile ingredient. They also have some amazing health benefits, such as a high amount of vitamins K and A. When not fasting, try adding in a lovely piece of wild-caught salmon for a bonus of healthy fats.

Heat the oil or fat in a small saucepan over medium heat. Add the onion and cook for 3 minutes, or until translucent.

Add the garlic, ginger, and cumin and cook for 30 seconds, or until fragrant.

Add the mustard greens, cauliflower, and broth and bring to a boil.

Once the liquid starts to boil, reduce the heat to low and simmer for 15 minutes, or until the vegetables are very tender. Add the coconut cream and spinach and cook for 30 seconds, or until the spinach is just wilted.

Blend the soup to a smooth consistency using a handheld blender. Season with salt and pepper to taste.

Ladle the soup into a warm bowl, scatter the nuts on top, and serve.

Serves: 1

1 Tbsp coconut oil or good-quality animal fat

¼ small onion, chopped

1 garlic clove, finely chopped

½ tsp finely grated ginger

½ tsp ground cumin

¾ cup roughly chopped mustard greens

¼ cup chopped cauliflower

1¾ cups Chicken Bone Broth (page 164; you can substitute beef broth or pork broth)

2 tsp coconut cream

4 to 6 leaves baby spinach

Sea salt and freshly ground black pepper

1 Tbsp roasted and chopped whole almond (activated if possible, i.e., soaked for 4 to 8 hours in salted water), to serve

NUTRITION INFORMATION

calories 308 | 24.6g total fat (14.7g saturated fat, 0.1g trans fat) | 3.9mg cholesterol
837.7mg sodium | 11g total carbohydrate (4.5g dietary fiber, 3.3g total sugars, -g added sugars)
13g protein | 0.1mcg vitamin D | 151.8mg calcium | 3.5mg iron | 837.7mg potassium

RADISH AND OKRA SOUP

Highly revered for its medicinal qualities, okra is said to be one of the greatest ingredients for people with diabetes to consume, and has been used for centuries in different parts of the world. Because of its mucilage-like properties, it makes its own release of a unique sliminess into dishes, adding thickness to gumbo and other stews and braises. Quickly pan-fried with some Indian spices, okra can be the star of the dish. When not fasting, this soup is great with the addition of some organic grass-fed and grass-finished beef meatballs too.

Serves: 1

1 Tbsp coconut oil or good-quality animal fat

¼ small onion, chopped

⅛ cup chopped celery

1 garlic clove, chopped

½ tsp cumin seeds

¼ tsp ground turmeric

Pinch of chili powder or cayenne pepper

2 okras, chopped

¼ cup diced daikon

¼ cup diced turnips

1¾ cups Chicken Bone Broth (page 164; you can substitute beef broth or pork broth)

3 Tbsp crushed whole peeled tomato

Sea salt and freshly ground black pepper

Cilantro sprigs, to serve

Heat the oil or fat in a small saucepan over medium heat. Add the onion and celery and cook for 3 minutes, or until translucent.

Add the garlic, cumin, turmeric, and chili powder and cook for 1 minute, or until fragrant.

Add the okra, daikon, turnips, broth, and tomatoes and bring to a boil. Reduce the heat to a gentle simmer and cook for 20 minutes. Season with salt and pepper to taste.

Blend the soup using a handheld blender until it's slightly smooth (some chunks of vegetables are fine), or you can leave the soup chunky.

Ladle the soup into a bowl, garnish with cilantro sprigs, and serve.

NUTRITION INFORMATION

calories 262.4 | 18.7g total fat (12.7g saturated fat, 0.1g trans fat) | 4.2mg cholesterol
836.2mg sodium | 12.9g total carbohydrate (3.5g dietary fiber, 5.5g total sugars, -g added sugars)
10.8g protein | 0.1mcg vitamin D | 97.7mg calcium | 2.9mg iron | 791.1mg potassium

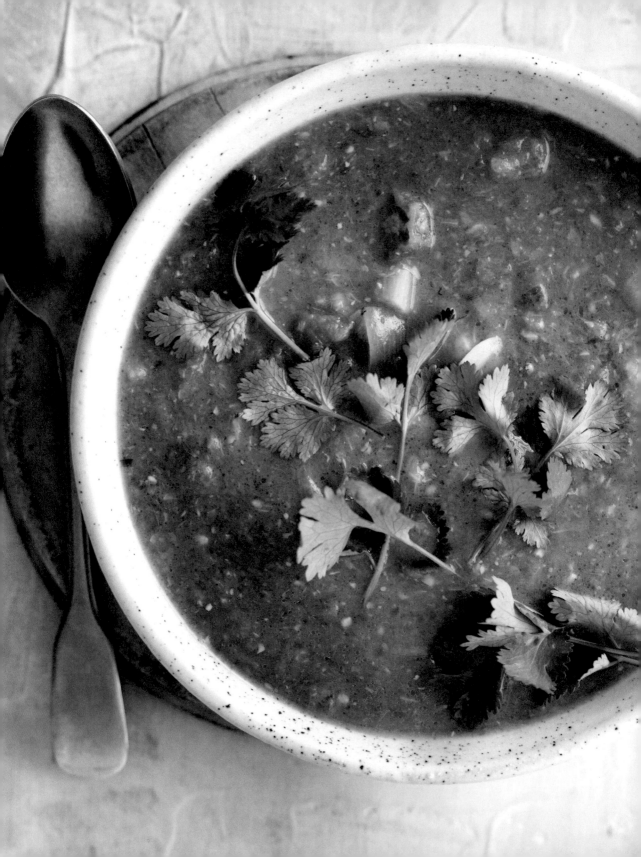

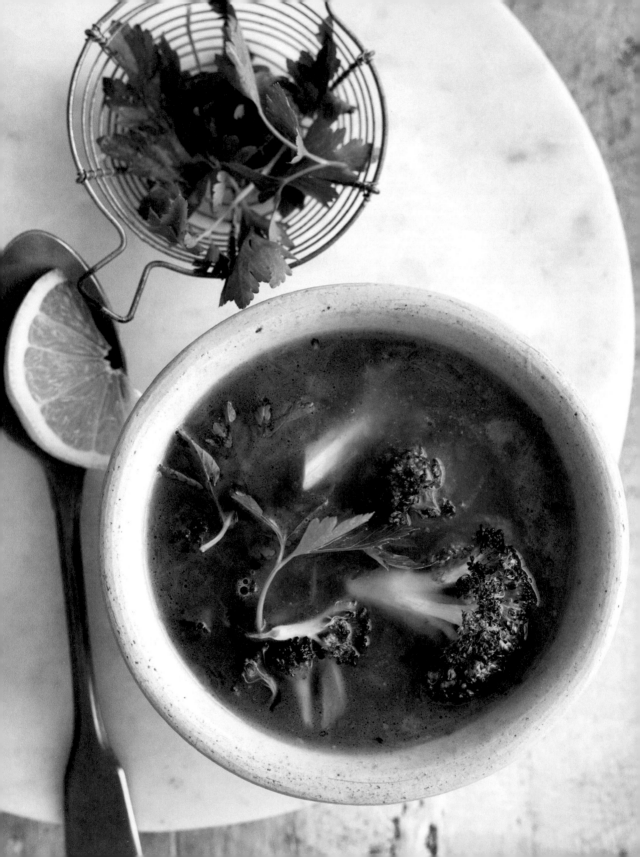

ROASTED BROCCOLI SOUP

When you roast vegetables you can extract more flavor from them, and this is where the magic happens from a taste and texture point of view. There is nothing wrong with steamed or boiled vegetables, and they do taste great, but you should experiment with roasting vegetables that you may have never thought about before. Vegetables such as cauliflower, broccoli, asparagus, mushrooms, brussels sprouts, celeriac, and so on all have unique flavor profiles that will surely surprise you.

Pete is a huge fan of using animal fats like duck fat, beef tallow from grass-fed and organic cattle, or coconut oil to coat the vegetables first. Next you'll want to season the vegetables well with good-quality salt prior to roasting to enhance the flavor. To add a twist and further enhance flavors, you can use aromatics like garlic and chili and herbs such as thyme. Here is a wonderful soup that takes broccoli to the next level and is truly a joy to eat.

Preheat the oven to 350°F.

Line a baking sheet with baking paper. Place the broccoli on the baking sheet and drizzle with 1 teaspoon of oil. Roast in the oven for 15 minutes, or until lightly golden and almost tender.

When the broccoli is almost finished roasting, heat a small saucepan with the remaining oil over medium heat. Add the onion and sauté for 3 minutes, or until translucent. Add the garlic and cook for 30 seconds, or until fragrant.

Add the roasted broccoli, cayenne pepper, thyme, and broth and stir to combine. Bring to a boil, cover with a lid, and reduce the heat to low, allowing the soup to gently simmer for 20 minutes, or until the vegetables are tender.

Add the lemon juice and tahini and season with salt and pepper to taste.

Ladle the soup into a warm bowl and garnish with fresh parsley.

Serves: 1

½ cup broccoli, broken into small florets

1 Tbsp coconut oil or good-quality animal fat, melted, divided

¼ small onion, chopped

2 garlic cloves, chopped

Pinch of cayenne pepper

¼ tsp chopped thyme leaves

1¾ cups Chicken Bone Broth (page 164; you can substitute beef broth or pork broth)

¼ tsp lemon juice

½ tsp hulled tahini

Sea salt and freshly ground black pepper

3 flat-leaf parsley sprigs, to garnish

NUTRITION INFORMATION

calories 259.5 | 19.9g total fat (12.9g saturated fat, 0.1g trans fat) | 4.2mg cholesterol
717.5mg sodium | 10.3g total carbohydrate (2.4g dietary fiber, 2.7g total sugars, -g added sugars)
1.3g protein | 0.1mcg vitamin D | 77mg calcium | 1.8mg iron | 605.3mg potassium

ROASTED BRUSSELS SPROUT
AND CAULIFLOWER SOUP

Brussels sprouts have become one of Pete's favorite vegetables to cook with over the past 10 years or so, which is awesome because they were the one vegetable that he didn't like as a child. It wasn't until he learned how to cook them properly that he began to appreciate them, as they really do have a wonderful earthy flavor that is developed with the correct cooking techniques.

Pete's favorite way to prepare them is by roasting them in either animal fat or coconut oil to extract their sweetness and give them a golden color. This soup could be the dish to turn the fussiest of brussels sprout eaters around; if you already love them, then you will adore this delicious offering.

Serves: 1

¼ small onion, chopped

1 garlic clove, finely chopped

⅓ cup cauliflower florets

1⅓ cups baby brussels sprouts, halved

1 Tbsp good-quality animal fat or coconut oil, melted

1¾ cups Beef or Chicken Bone Broth (pages 163 and 164)

Sea salt and freshly ground black pepper

Chopped parsley for garnish

A couple of splashes of truffle oil or extra-virgin olive oil (optional)

Preheat the oven to 400°F.

Place all the vegetables in a bowl, add the fat, and toss to coat. Spread the vegetables on a baking sheet and roast them in the oven for 15 to 20 minutes (tossing halfway), until lightly golden.

Reserve 8 of the roasted brussels sprout halves and set them aside.

Transfer the remaining roasted vegetables from the sheet into a saucepan. Pour in the broth and bring to a boil. Turn the heat down to low and gently simmer for 20 minutes, or until the vegetables are very tender.

Blend the soup with a handheld blender until smooth, then season with salt and pepper to taste.

Add the reserved brussels sprouts to the soup and simmer for 1 minute, until heated through.

Ladle the soup into a bowl, sprinkle with some chopped parsley, and drizzle with a couple of splashes of truffle oil (if using).

NUTRITION INFORMATION

calories 339.3 | 25.4g total fat (18.4g saturated fat, 0.1g trans fat) | 4.2mg cholesterol
1758.7mg sodium | 16.9g total carbohydrate (5.7g dietary fiber, 4.8g total sugars, -g added sugars)
13.7g protein | 0.1mcg vitamin D | 88.9mg calcium | 2.8mg iron | 954.4mg potassium

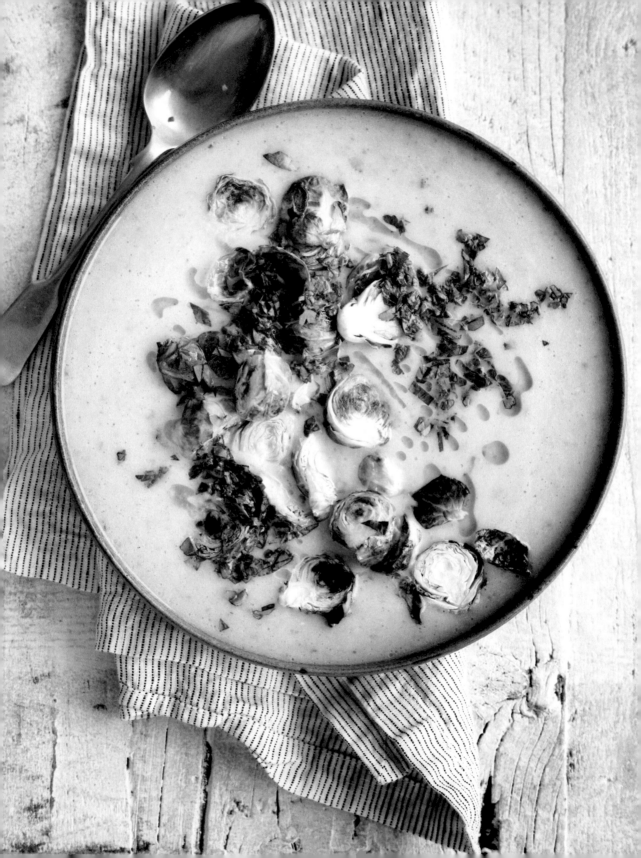

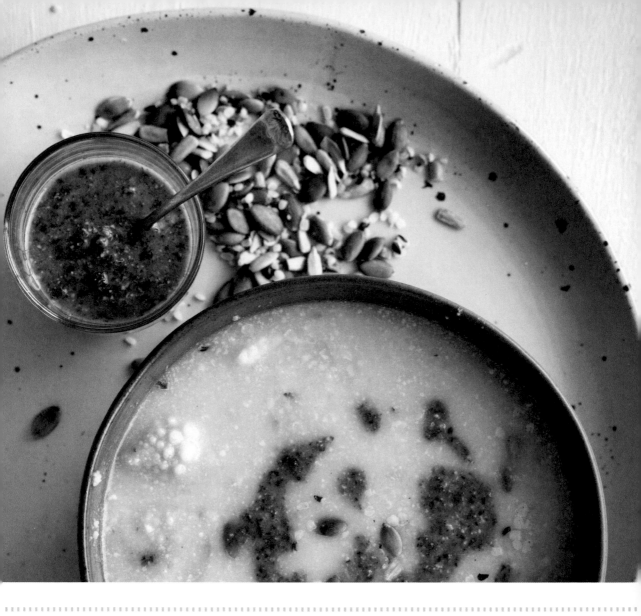

PESTO

To make the pesto, place all the ingredients in a bowl and mix well to combine. Season with salt and pepper to taste.

1 Tbsp finely chopped mint

2 tsp finely chopped walnuts

1 Tbsp olive oil

2 tsp lemon juice

Sea salt and freshly ground black pepper, to taste

ROMANESCO SOUP WITH PESTO

The very psychedelic-looking Romanesco vegetable that has a wondrous fractal forma-tion has become more and more popular over the past decade, and not only because of its appearance but because of its delicious flavor. It is very similar to cauliflower but has a nuttier flavor that is a little deeper and richer, and it can be eaten raw, slightly cooked, or cooked all the way through. With this soup, Pete kept it beautiful and creamy, and added a luscious herb oil and toasted seeds to elevate the dish to be a star of the dinner table. When you're not fast-ing, feel free to add seared scallops, poached white-flesh wild fish, or organic chicken.

To make the soup, melt the oil in a small saucepan over medium heat. Add the onion and garlic and cook for 3 minutes, or until softened. Stir in the Romanesco and broth and bring to a boil. Cover, reduce the heat to low, and simmer for 20 minutes, or until the Romanesco is tender.

Blend the soup with a handheld blender until almost smooth, keeping it slightly chunky. Season with salt and pepper to taste.

Ladle the soup into a warm bowl, drizzle some pesto over the top, and finish with some seeds.

NOTE: If Romanesco is not available, you can substitute cauliflower, broccoli, or both.

Serves: 1

1 Tbsp coconut oil or good-quality animal fat

¼ small onion, chopped

1 garlic clove, finely chopped

1⅓ cups Romanesco broccoli, cut into small florets (see note)

1¾ cups Chicken Bone Broth (page 164; you can substitute beef broth or pork broth)

Salt and freshly ground black pepper

Pesto (page 110)

1 Tbsp pumpkin seeds and sunflower seeds, to serve

NUTRITION INFORMATION

calories 493.2 | 43.1g total fat (15.8g saturated fat, 0.1g trans fat) | 4.2mg cholesterol
731mg sodium | 14.2g total carbohydrate (4.9g dietary fiber, 3.7g total sugars, -g added sugars)
16.6g protein | 0.1mcg vitamin D | 75.6mg calcium | 2.8mg iron | 523.8mg potassium

SIMPLE PHO

One of Pete's all-time favorite Vietnamese dishes is the ever-addictive pho (pronounced *fuh*), which is a concoction of animal bones simmering slowly away in a large pot with herbs and spices. It takes an already delicious base and turns it into something memorable for all the right reasons. Here is a very quick and easy version that you can make in a matter of minutes that will enliven any day of the week. When not fasting, try adding some wild-caught seafood, such as mussels or wild salmon, or organic chicken or beef.

Serves: 1

1 Tbsp coconut oil or good-quality animal fat

¼ small onion, sliced

1 garlic clove, finely chopped

1 tsp finely grated ginger

1¾ cups Beef Bone Broth (page 163)

¼ tsp ground coriander seeds

1 cinnamon stick

2 star anise pods

1 pinch of ground cloves

2 tsp fish sauce

About half a spring onion (green part only), julienned

⅔ cup spiralized zucchini

1 tsp finely chopped red chili

Lemon or lime juice, to taste

Lemon or lime wedge, to serve

1 small handful Thai basil or cilantro, for garnish

Heat the oil or fat in a small frying pan over medium heat. Add the onion and cook for 3 minutes, or until translucent. Add the garlic and ginger and cook for 30 seconds, or until fragrant.

Add the broth, coriander, cinnamon, star anise, cloves, and fish sauce. Bring to a boil, then reduce the heat to low. Cover and gently simmer for 25 minutes.

Add the spring onion and spiralized zucchini and simmer for 30 seconds. Remove and discard the cinnamon and star anise.

Ladle the pho into a warm bowl. Add some chili and a squeeze of lemon or lime juice to taste—and, if needed, add a little more fish sauce. To finish, garnish with some Thai basil.

NUTRITION INFORMATION

calories 193.5 | 14g total fat (11.3g saturated fat, 0g trans fat) | 0mg cholesterol
1714.1mg sodium | 9g total carbohydrate (3.1g dietary fiber, 4.2g total sugars, -g added sugars)
10g protein | 0mcg vitamin D | 103.9mg calcium | 2.6mg iron | 1055.7mg potassium

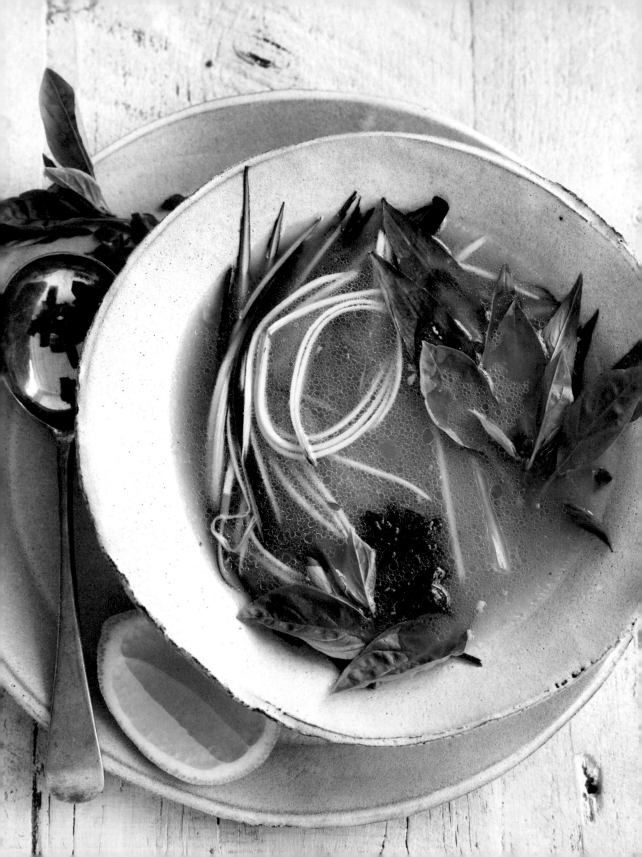

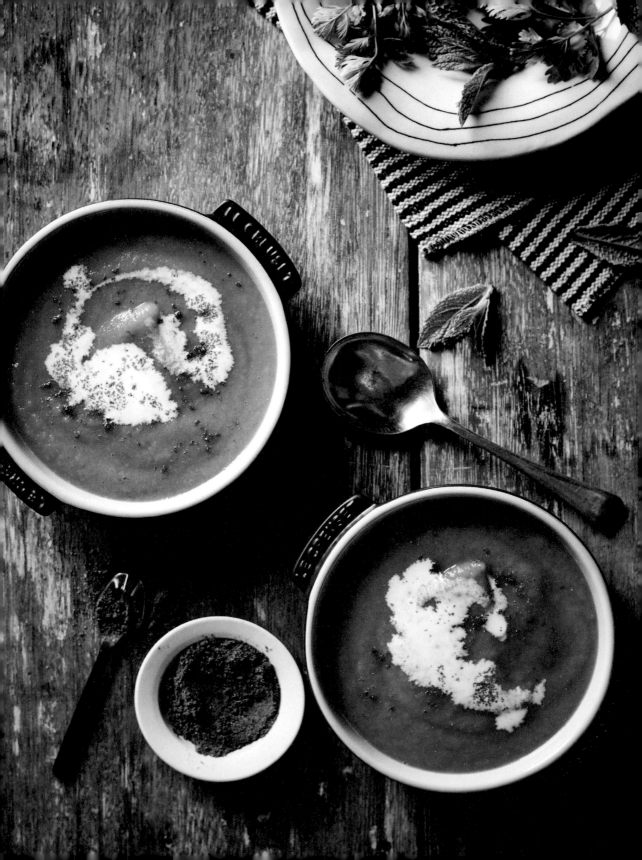

SPICED SQUASH SOUP

Who doesn't love a bowl of luscious, lightly spiced squash soup on a cold winter's night? Squash soup tends to tick a lot of boxes for families—it is super-cheap, nutritious, pleasing to all tastebuds, and perfect for leftovers the next day. Try packing it as a school lunch in a thermos or enjoying it for a quick breakfast with a poached egg or some leftover roasted chicken, pork, or lamb on top.

Heat the oil or fat in a large saucepan over medium heat. Add the squash, carrot, onion, and garlic and sauté, stirring occasionally, for about 10 minutes, until the onion is translucent.

Add the broth, ginger, Ras el Hanout, cumin, saffron, and chili flakes, if using. Reduce the heat, cover, and simmer, stirring occasionally, for about 30 minutes, or until the carrot and squash are tender.

Add the coconut cream and puree the soup using a handheld blender. Season to taste with salt and pepper.

Ladle the soup into bowls, drizzle with a little extra coconut cream, and top with some cilantro and mint leaves and chili powder.

NOTE: Ras el Hanout is a North African spice mix that consists of more than 12 spices. Pete likes to use Ras el Hanout from Herbie's Spices in this recipe.

Serves: 4

3 Tbsp coconut oil or good-quality animal fat

1½ lb butternut squash (or any other squash variety), peeled and diced

1 carrot, diced

1 large onion, finely chopped

4 garlic cloves, crushed

5½ cups Chicken Bone Broth or Vegetable Broth (pages 164 and 172)

1½ Tbsp finely grated ginger

1½ Tbsp Ras el Hanout (see note)

1½ tsp ground cumin

6 saffron threads

1 tsp dried chili flakes (optional)

1 cup coconut cream, plus extra to serve

Sea salt and freshly ground black pepper

Cilantro and mint leaves, to serve

Chili powder, to serve

NUTRITION INFORMATION

calories 382.4 | 30.1g total fat (24g saturated fat, 0.1g trans fat) | 3.3mg cholesterol
460.9mg sodium | 19.9g total carbohydrate (2g dietary fiber, 8.9g total sugars, -g added sugars)
10.6g protein | 0.1mcg vitamin D | 69.7mg calcium | 2.3mg iron | 1137.4mg potassium

SPROUTED MUNG BEAN SOUP

This recipe is the one that started this whole book; it's why I contacted Pete to see if he would collaborate with me on a fasting cookbook. I wanted to include sprouted mung beans and asked if Pete could make a soup that had them as the star, but that also fit into the formula for fasting. And, of course, it had to be absolutely delicious. So here is the first recipe we created and I have to say, it's absolutely delicious!

Serves: 1

1 Tbsp coconut oil or good-quality animal fat

¼ onion, chopped

1 garlic clove, finely chopped

¼ tsp finely grated ginger

¼ tsp ground turmeric

½ tsp ground cumin

½ cup sprouted mung beans

1¾ cups Beef or Chicken Bone Broth (pages 163 and 164)

¼ cup baby spinach

¼ tsp lemon juice, or more to taste

Sea salt and freshly ground black pepper

Heat the oil or fat in a small saucepan over medium heat. Add the onion and cook for 3 minutes, or until translucent. Add the garlic, ginger, turmeric, and cumin and cook for 30 seconds, or until fragrant.

Add the mung beans and broth. Bring to a simmer, then reduce the heat to low and gently simmer for 20 minutes.

Add the spinach and cook for 30 seconds, or until wilted. Mix in the lemon juice and season with salt and pepper to taste.

NUTRITION INFORMATION

calories 247.4 | 18.7g total fat (12.7g saturated fat, 0.1g trans fat) | 4.2mg cholesterol
2907.3mg sodium | 9.8g total carbohydrate (2.2g dietary fiber, 2.9g total sugars, -g added sugars)
11.6g protein | 0.1mcg vitamin D | 70.9mg calcium | 3.1mg iron | 611.3mg potassium

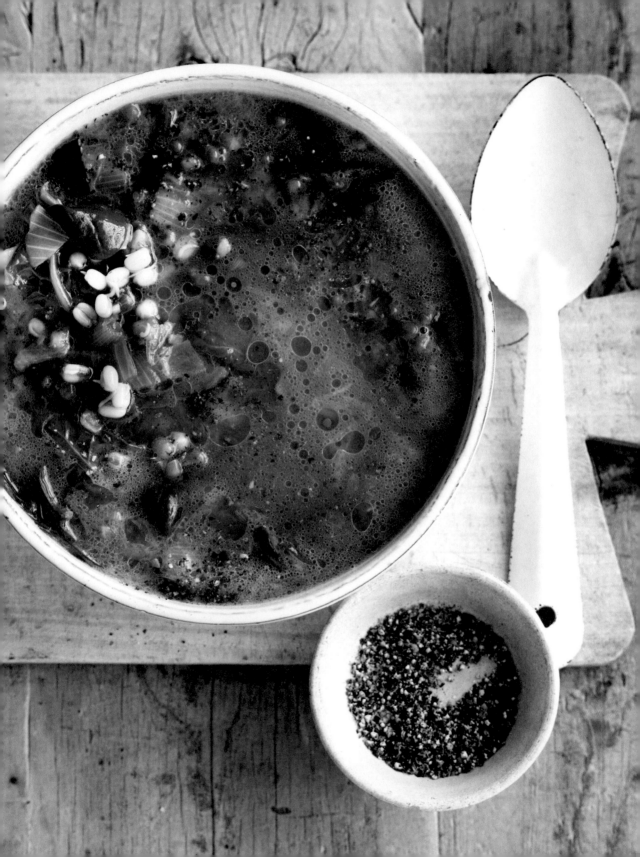

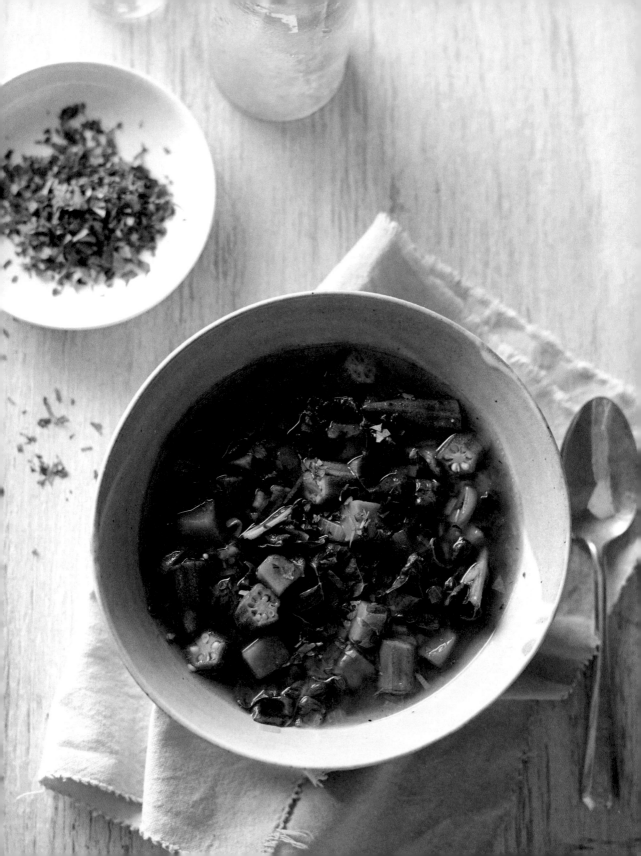

WARMING VEGETABLE SOUP

This is a soup I love to make at home, changing the veggies depending on the availability of the season. It is a simple soup to digest and is great for breakfast. You could, of course, add some protein; try leftover roasted chicken, braised lamb shanks or oxtail, or, for a seafood hit, some prawns or wild salmon.

Heat the oil or fat in a large saucepan over low heat. Add the onion and a sprinkle of salt and cook slowly, stirring occasionally, for about 15 minutes, or until the onion is soft and golden.

Add the garlic, ginger, and leek and cook for 1 minute. Stir in the sweet potato, broth, and 1 teaspoon of the salt and bring to a boil. Reduce the heat, add the kale and okra, and simmer for 15 minutes. You can either puree the soup or leave it chunky.

Stir 2 teaspoons of the lemon juice into the soup. Add the parsley and a few grinds of pepper to taste. Add more salt or lemon juice to taste. Spoon into bowls and serve.

Serves: 6

2 Tbsp coconut oil

1 large yellow onion, chopped

1½ tsp sea salt, divided, plus more to taste

2 garlic cloves, chopped

3 Tbsp chopped ginger, plus more to taste

½ large leek (white and light green parts only), sliced

½ small sweet potato, diced

4 cups Chicken Bone Broth or Vegetable Broth (pages 164 and 172)

½ bunch kale (about ½ pound), roughly chopped

¼ lb okra, cut into 1-inch pieces

2 to 4 tsp lemon juice

1 handful flat-leaf parsley leaves, chopped

Freshly ground black pepper

NUTRITION INFORMATION
calories 156.6 | 11.3g total fat (8.1g saturated fat, 0g trans fat) | 1.8mg cholesterol
697.9mg sodium | 9.5g total carbohydrate (2.2g dietary fiber, 2.8g total sugars, -g added sugars)
5.6g protein | 0.1mcg vitamin D | 72.2mg calcium | 1.5mg iron | 460.9mg potassium

WATERCRESS, CABBAGE, AND SHIITAKE SOUP

This recipe just screams out to be eaten at any time of the year and is one of Pete's all-time favorites in this book. The reason he loves it so much is because chefs are always striving for simplicity—where less is more, so that the dishes they create are not overcomplicated. That same philosophy can be carried through to many aspects of our lives. Here he took a wonderful broth as the base, then added some mushrooms for that umami flavor, and also some health-boosting watercress. I encourage you to try this soup, and when you're not fasting, experiment by adding an organic egg, free-range organic duck, organic chicken, or pasture-raised organic slow-cooked pork belly.

Serves: 1

1 Tbsp coconut oil or good-quality animal fat

½ small carrot, sliced

1 garlic clove, finely chopped

½ spring onion (white part only), thinly sliced

1 large leaf green cabbage, shredded

⅛ cup thinly sliced shiitake mushroom

1¾ cups Chicken Bone Broth (page 164; you can substitute beef broth or pork broth)

½ tsp finely grated ginger

1 tsp tamari or coconut aminos

½ tsp toasted sesame oil

¼ tsp fish sauce

4 sprigs fresh watercress

Heat the oil or fat in a saucepan over medium heat. Add the carrot, garlic, and onion and cook for 3 minutes, until slightly softened and starting to color.

Add the cabbage, shiitake, broth, ginger, tamari, sesame oil, and fish sauce and stir well. Bring to a boil, then turn down the heat to low and gently simmer for 20 minutes, or until the vegetables are tender.

Add the watercress and simmer for 30 seconds, or until wilted. Season with a little salt or more fish sauce to taste.

Ladle the broth into a bowl and serve.

NUTRITION INFORMATION

calories 263 | 20.7g total fat (13g saturated fat, 0.1g trans fat) | 4.2mg cholesterol
1029.5mg sodium | 9.3g total carbohydrate (2.2g dietary fiber, 3.7g total sugars, -g added sugars)
10.8g protein | 0.2mcg vitamin D | 62.8mg calcium | 1.4mg iron | 602.5mg potassium

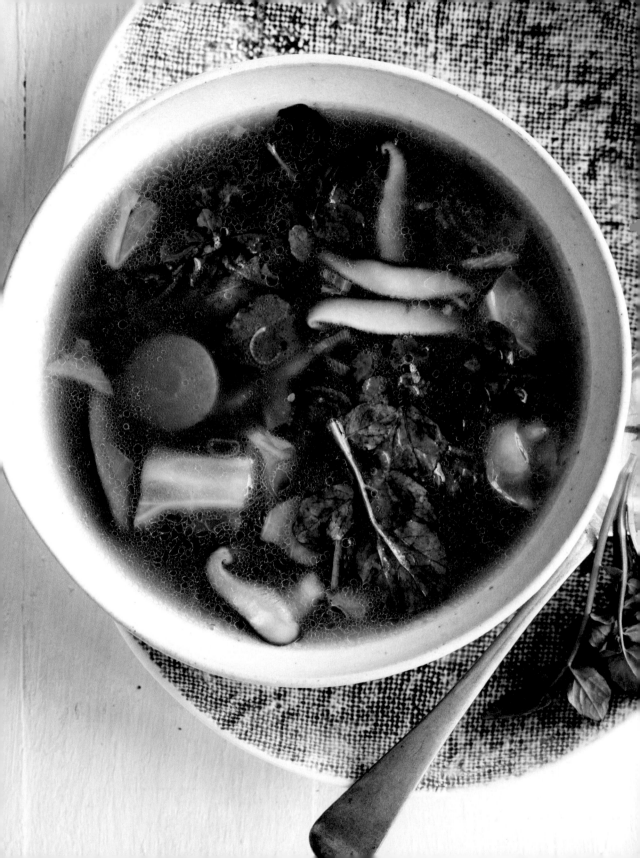

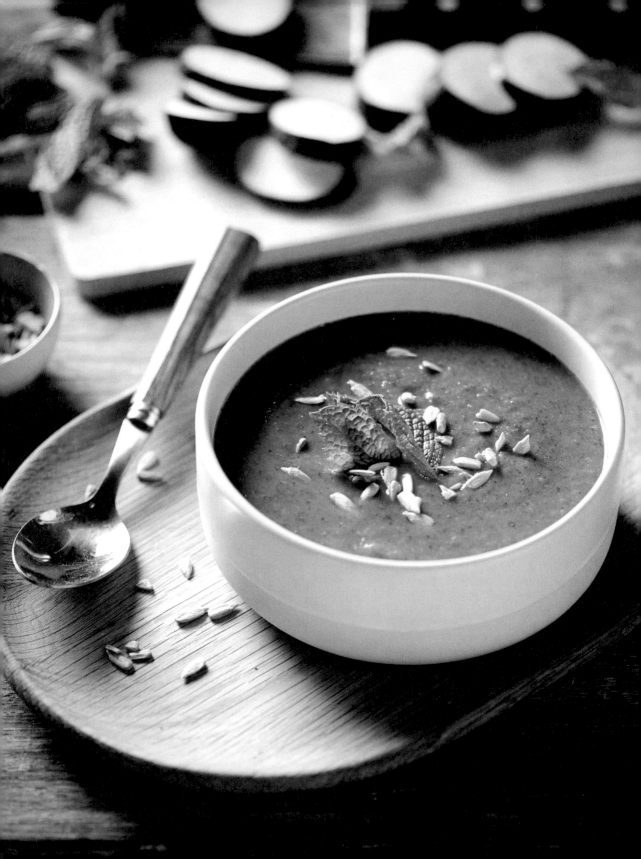

ZUCCHINI SOUP
WITH FRESH MINT

Try this nourishing soup in the summertime when zucchinis are overtaking your garden, or when you see them on sale at your local farmers market or supermarket. The addition of mint is a masterstroke; and if you want to take your soup to another level, add some chili flakes and any type of seafood.

Heat the oil in a large saucepan over medium heat. Add the onion and garlic and sauté for a few minutes, until the onion is translucent.

Add the zucchini to the pan and cook for 5 minutes, or until softened. Add the cauliflower and broth and bring to a boil. Reduce the heat to low, cover, and simmer for 20 minutes, or until the cauliflower is tender.

Stir the spinach into the soup, then puree with a handheld blender until smooth. Add more hot broth as needed if the soup is too thick. Season with salt and pepper. Serve topped with some mint leaves and sunflower seeds.

Serves: 6

3 Tbsp coconut oil

1 onion, chopped

3 garlic cloves, chopped

2 medium zucchinis, chopped

½ lb cauliflower florets

5½ cups Chicken Bone Broth (page 164), plus extra hot broth if needed

2 handfuls baby spinach leaves

Sea salt and freshly ground white pepper

Mint leaves, to serve

Sunflower seeds, to serve

NUTRITION INFORMATION
calories 147.5 | 10.3g total fat (6.5g saturated fat, 0g trans fat) | 2.2mg cholesterol
418.8mg sodium | 7.7g total carbohydrate (2.3g dietary fiber, 3.4g total sugars, -g added sugars)
7g protein | 0.1mcg vitamin D | 60.7mg calcium | 1.8mg iron | 628mg potassium

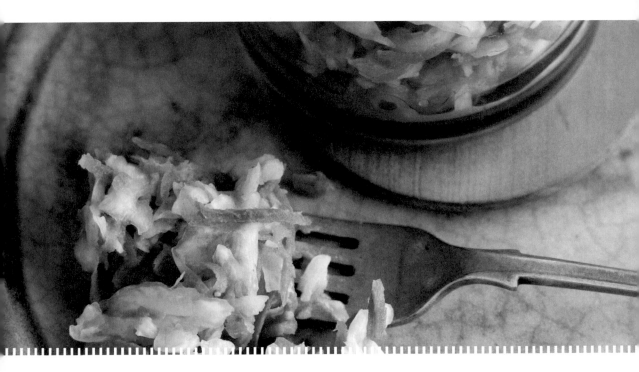

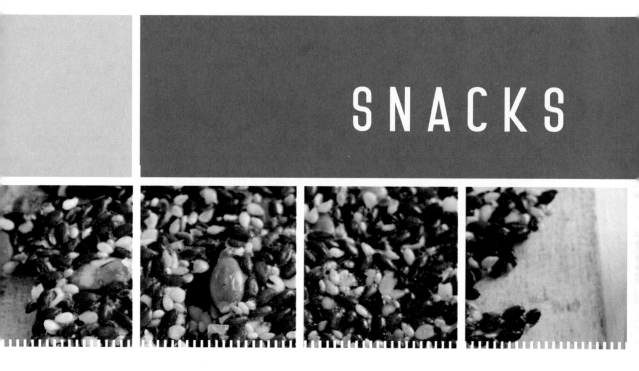

SNACKS

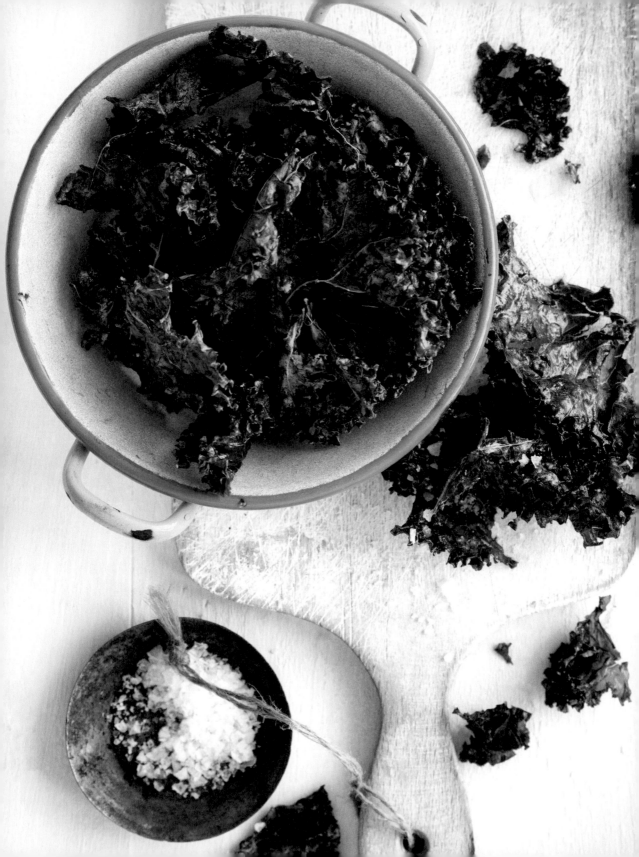

KALE CHIPS

Pete has been making kale chips for the past decade or so and they are always devoured as soon as they hit the serving platter (if they make it that far!). When the kale is slowly cooked and coated in healthy fats as well as good-quality salt and spices, the flavor and texture can become addictive. You can either eat kale chips on their own or place some on top of your soups, broths, or meals for that little something extra. And the good news is that even kids love them.

Preheat the oven to 250°F.

Line a baking sheet with parchment paper.

Wash the kale thoroughly in cold water and pat dry.

Remove and discard the tough central stems, then cut the leaves into smaller pieces.

Toss the kale with some coconut oil, spice (if using), and salt in a large bowl. (Go easy on the salt; a little goes a long way.) Spread the kale on the baking sheet in a single layer; do not overcrowd. Use more than one baking sheet, if needed. Roast the kale for 35 to 40 minutes, until crispy.

Serve immediately or store in an airtight container in the pantry for up to 2 weeks.

Serves: 2

1 bunch kale (about ¾ pound)

1 Tbsp coconut oil, melted

½ tsp of your favorite spice (such as curry powder, paprika, ground cumin, or ground turmeric) (optional)

Sea salt

NUTRITION INFORMATION
calories 39.1 | 3.6g total fat (2.8g saturated fat, 0g trans fat) | 0mg cholesterol
152.4mg sodium | 1.5g total carbohydrate (0.7g dietary fiber, 0.4g total sugars, -g added sugars)
0.7g protein | 0mcg vitamin D | 25.7mg calcium | 0.3mg iron | 81.6mg potassium

SPICY
PUMPKIN SEED "POPCORN"

Spiced seeds are among the yummiest snacks around. Not only are they delicious to eat by themselves, but they are also an awesome topping to the broths and soups in this book. But don't stop there as they can add a wonderful texture and flavor to salads, grilled or steamed fish, and even egg and vegetable dishes. Play with different spices and seeds to create different flavor profiles.

Serves: 2

1 Tbsp coconut oil

1½ tsp cumin seeds

1 cup pumpkin seeds

¼ tsp chili flakes

Sea salt

Heat the oil in a frying pan over medium-high heat. Add the cumin seeds and pumpkin seeds and cook, stirring frequently, for 2½ to 3 minutes, or until the seeds are toasted. (You will hear them start to pop). Add the chili flakes, sprinkle with a good pinch of salt, and enjoy while warm.

NUTRITION INFORMATION
calories 177.1 | 15.8g total fat (5g saturated fat, 0g trans fat) | 0mg cholesterol
152.4mg sodium | 4.1g total carbohydrate (1.7g dietary fiber, 0.4g total sugars, -g added sugars)
7.6g protein | 0mcg vitamin D | 20.5mg calcium | 2.5mg iron | 211.9mg potassium

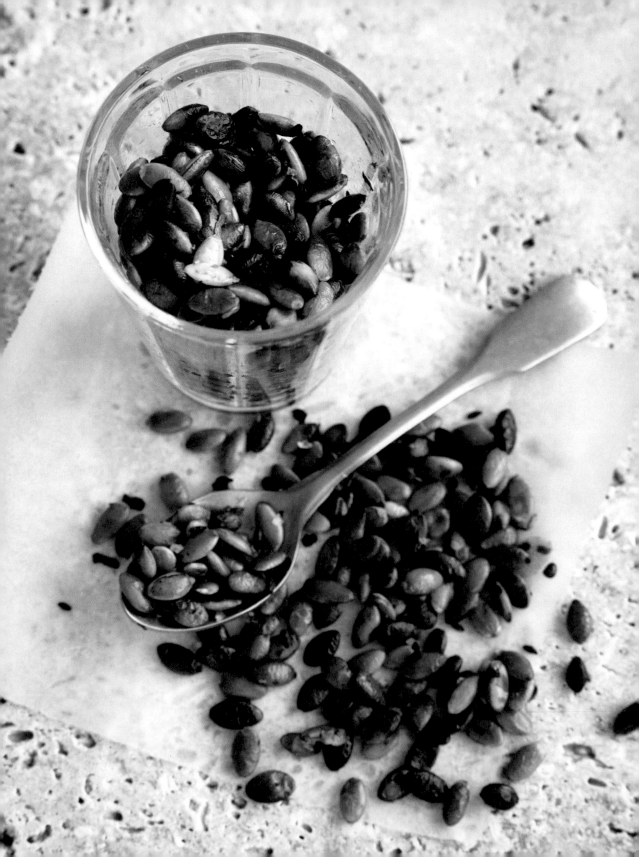

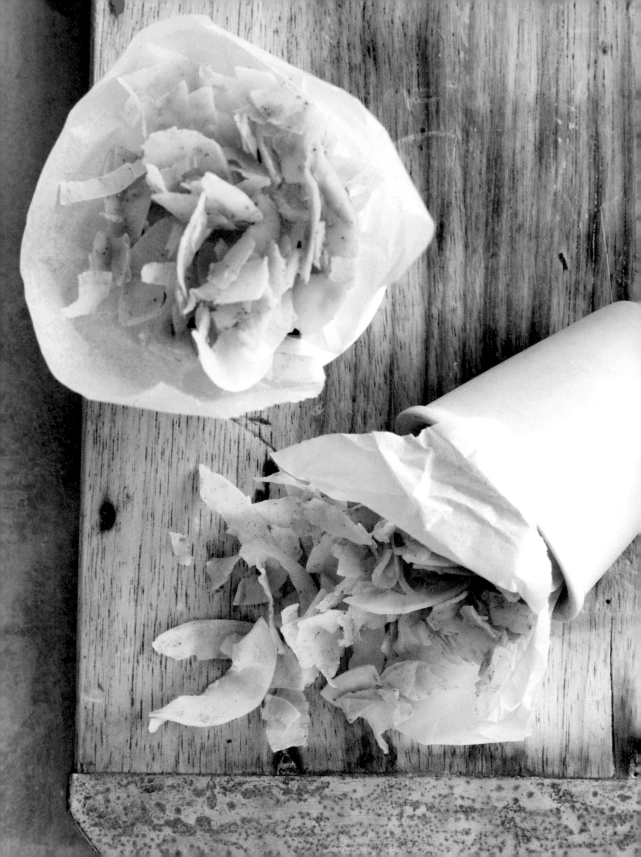

TURMERIC AND GINGER COCONUT CHIPS

When coming up with recipes for this book, I insisted that we have additions to the soups and broths as well as treats and snacks, so you can have fun when you are on the fast. Pete enjoyed coming up with different recipes that would be pleasant and tasty and still fit in with the requirements of my philosophy. So here are our turmeric-and-ginger-spiced coconut chips. They are utterly delicious.

Preheat the oven to 300°F.

Line a baking sheet with parchment paper.

Place the coconut oil, turmeric, ginger, and honey in a bowl and stir to combine. Sprinkle with some salt.

Add the coconut chips and toss gently until the coconut is well coated.

Spread the coconut over the prepared sheet in a single layer and bake, stirring gently every 5 minutes or so, for 15 to 20 minutes, or until lightly golden. Keep a close eye on the coconut after 10 minutes as it can burn quickly.

Remove the sheet from the oven and allow the coconut to cool completely before serving. Store in an airtight container in the pantry for up to 2 weeks.

Serves: 3 to 4

2 Tbsp coconut oil

1 tsp ground turmeric

1 tsp ground ginger

2 tsp raw honey

Pinch of sea salt

1⅓ cups coconut chips

NUTRITION INFORMATION
calories 220.7 | 21.3g total fat (18.5g saturated fat, 0g trans fat) | 0mg cholesterol
154.8mg sodium | 8.3g total carbohydrate (3.9g dietary fiber, 3.7g total sugars, -g added sugars)
1.7g protein | 0mcg vitamin D | 8.1mg calcium | 1.3mg iron | 144.2mg potassium

TURMERIC KRAUT

Pete wanted to take the humble but powerful sauerkraut and upgrade it to a nutritional powerhouse with the addition of turmeric. Many people may not realize that when turmeric is fermented, not only does it become more bioavailable to the body, but its potency increases. So if you want more bioavailable turmeric and probiotic goodness in your diet, then this is for you!

Makes: 1 quart

4½ cups cabbage (you can use green or red, or a mixture of the two)

3 medium carrots, grated

2 Tbsp finely grated ginger

3 tsp ground turmeric

2 tsp caraway seeds

2 Tbsp fine Himalayan or sea salt

You will need a 1-quart preserving jar with an airlock lid for this recipe. Wash the jar and all the utensils you will be using in very hot water or run them through a hot rinse cycle in the dishwasher.

Remove the outer leaves of the cabbage. Choose 1 of the outer leaves, wash it well, and set it aside. Shred the remainder of the cabbage in a food processor, or slice it by hand.

Combine the grated carrot, shredded cabbage, ginger, turmeric, and caraway seeds in a bowl, then sprinkle with the salt. Massage the ingredients together for 10 minutes to release some liquid.

Fill the prepared jar with the cabbage mixture, pressing down firmly with a large spoon or potato masher to remove any air pockets. Leave ¾ inch of room free at the top. The vegetables should be completely submerged in the liquid; add some filtered water if necessary.

Take the clean cabbage leaf, fold it up to fit in the jar, and place it on top of the cabbage mixture. Add a small glass weight (a shot glass is ideal) to keep everything submerged. Close the lid, then wrap a tea towel around the side of the jar to block out any light.

Store in a dark place with a temperature of 60° to 75°F for 12 to 14 days. (Place the jar in a cooler to maintain a more consistent temperature.) Different vegetables have different culturing times and the warmer it is, the shorter the time needed. The longer you leave the jar, the higher the level of good bacteria and the tangier the flavor.

NUTRITION INFORMATION

calories 14.3 | 0.1g total fat (0g saturated fat, 0g trans fat) | 0mg cholesterol
714mg sodium | 3.2g total carbohydrate (1.2g dietary fiber, 1.5g total sugars, -g added sugars)
0.6g protein | 0mcg vitamin D | 19.3mg calcium | 0.5mg iron | 98.3mg potassium

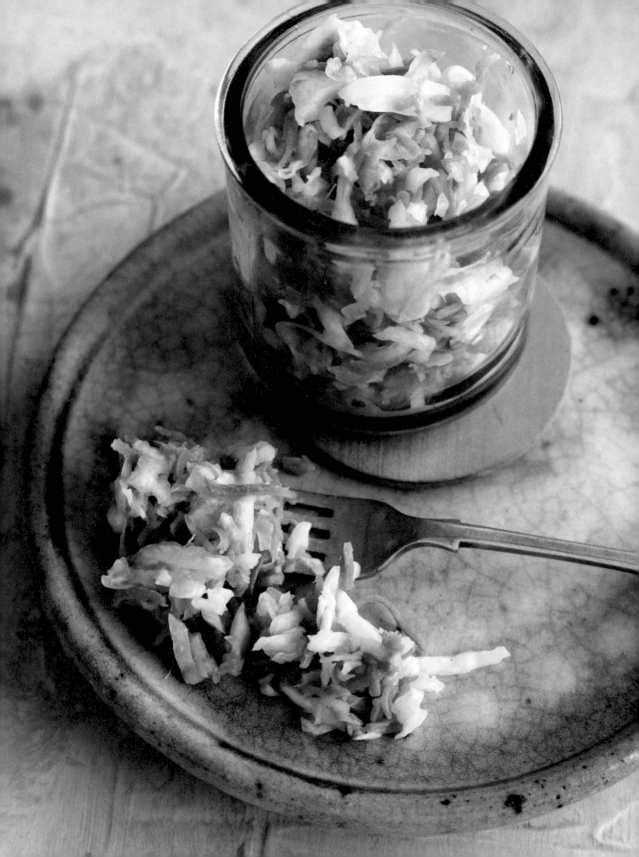

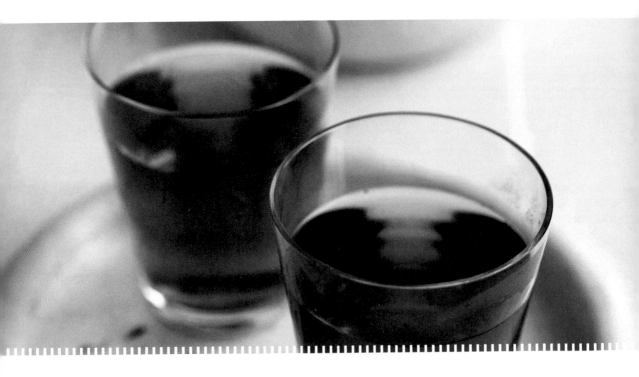

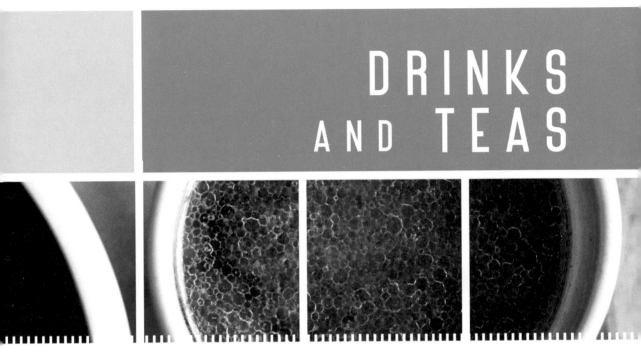

DRINKS
AND TEAS

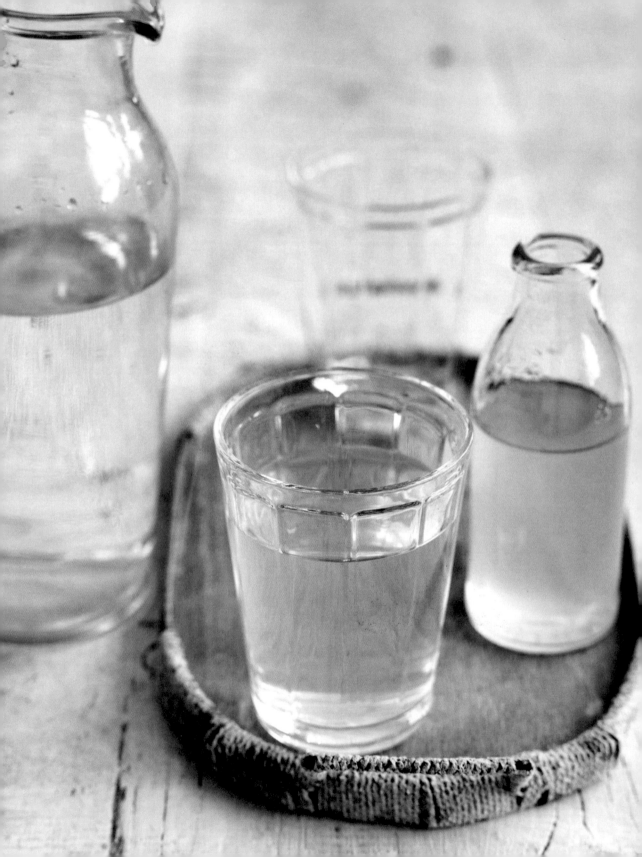

APPLE CIDER VINEGAR WATER

This simple approach of popping a little organic apple cider vinegar with its mother in some good-quality water can never be underestimated as a great way to wake up and enliven your system in the morning; it is very inexpensive and you'll actually start to crave that sharpness after making it part of your daily routine. As an alternative, you could use some fresh organic lemon or organic lime juice instead.

Stir the water and apple cider vinegar together and drink.

Serves: 1

2 cups filtered water, room temperature

2 tsp apple cider vinegar

NUTRITION INFORMATION

calories 2.1 | 0g total fat (0g saturated fat, 0g trans fat) | 0mg cholesterol
19.5mg sodium | 0.1g total carbohydrate (0g dietary fiber, 0g total sugars, -g added sugars)
0g protein | 0mcg vitamin D | 14.9mg calcium | 0mg iron | 7.3mg potassium

BEEF BONE BROTH TEA

This is the ultimate multivitamin for our bodies and it is so cheap and delicious, and also easy to make. Bone broth contains collagen, gelatin, glucosamine, calcium, magnesium, potassium, and a whole lot more, including good healthy fats. Try making about 5 quarts of broth a week, and drink it straight or use it for the base of soups and other meals. Beef broth can be strong for some, so you may want to start with chicken broth instead.

Serves: 1

1½ cups Beef Bone Broth

1 Tbsp coconut oil or good-quality animal fat

1 to 2 pinches of sea salt, to taste

½ tsp lemon juice or apple cider vinegar (optional)

Heat the broth in a saucepan until just simmering and stir in the oil. Add the salt and lemon juice (if using) to taste.

Pour the broth into a mug and serve.

NUTRITION INFORMATION

calories 20.6 | 0g total fat (0g saturated fat, 0g trans fat) | 0mg cholesterol
475.7mg sodium | 0.6g total carbohydrate (0g dietary fiber, 0.5g total sugars, -g added sugars)
4.7g protein | 0mcg vitamin D | 14.7mg calcium | 0.8mg iron | 442.8mg potassium

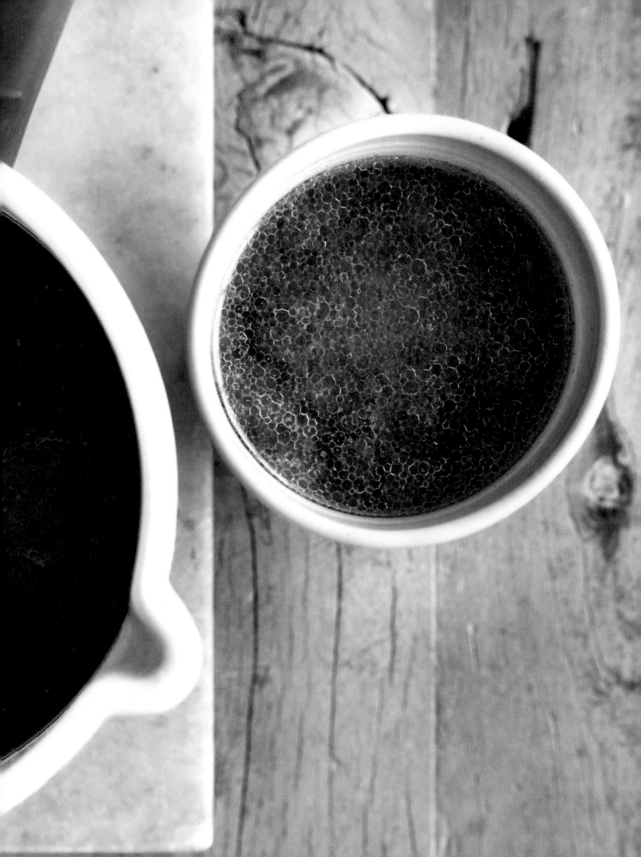

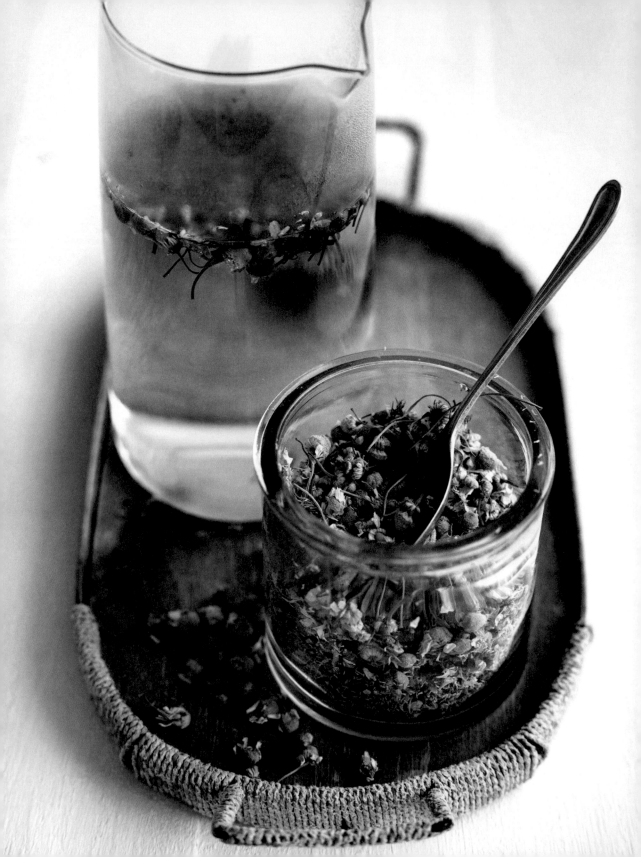

CHAMOMILE TEA

Pete is a huge fan of herbal tea and chamomile, in particular. This tea is a great nightcap at the end of dinner. Chamomile has a very calming effect on the nervous system and it helps to gently prepare you for sleep. Of course you can also can use it in the daytime when stressful situations arise.

Fill a mug with boiling water.

Stir in the chamomile and allow to infuse for 3 minutes. Strain and serve.

Serves: 1

2 tsp dried chamomile

NUTRITION INFORMATION

calories 2.4 | 0g total fat (0g saturated fat, 0g trans fat) | 0mg cholesterol
2.4mg sodium | 0.5g total carbohydrate (0g dietary fiber, 0g total sugars, -g added sugars)
0g protein | 0mcg vitamin D | 4.7mg calcium | 0.2mg iron | 21.3mg potassium

CHICORY TEA

Chicory tea is a wonderful alternative to caffeinated coffee or black tea, and has been used for centuries as a medicinal ingredient. Chicory has anti-inflammatory properties, as well as aiding in gut health and helping with constipation. It has even shown promising signs of helping those with osteoporosis.

Serves: 1

2 tsp dried chicory root

Fill a mug with boiling water.

Stir in the dried chicory root and leave to infuse for 3 minutes. Strain and serve.

NUTRITION INFORMATION
calories 6.7 | 0g total fat (0g saturated fat, 0g trans fat) | 0mg cholesterol
14.2mg sodium | 1.6g total carbohydrate (0.1g dietary fiber, 0.8g total sugars, -g added sugars)
0.1g protein | 0mcg vitamin D | 10.9mg calcium | 0.1mg iron | 27.1mg potassium

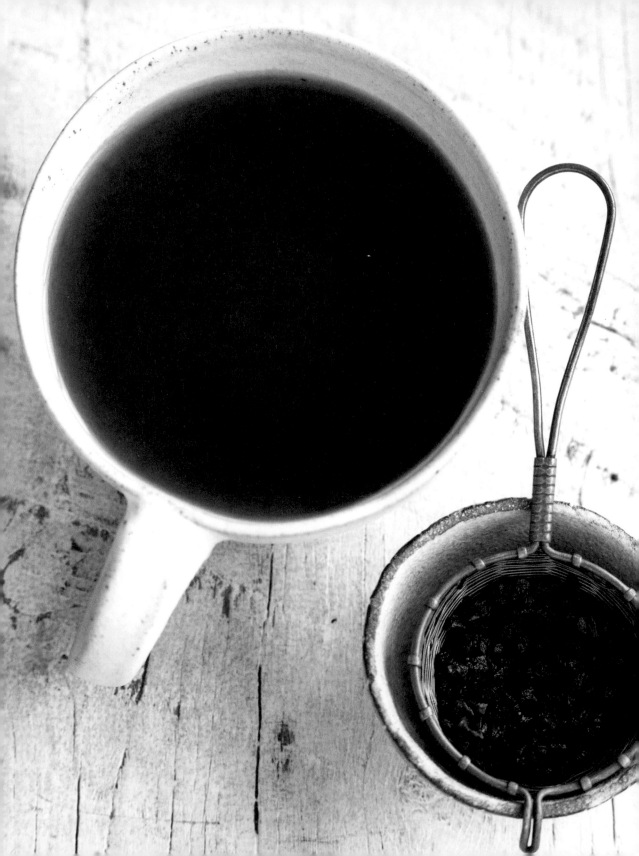

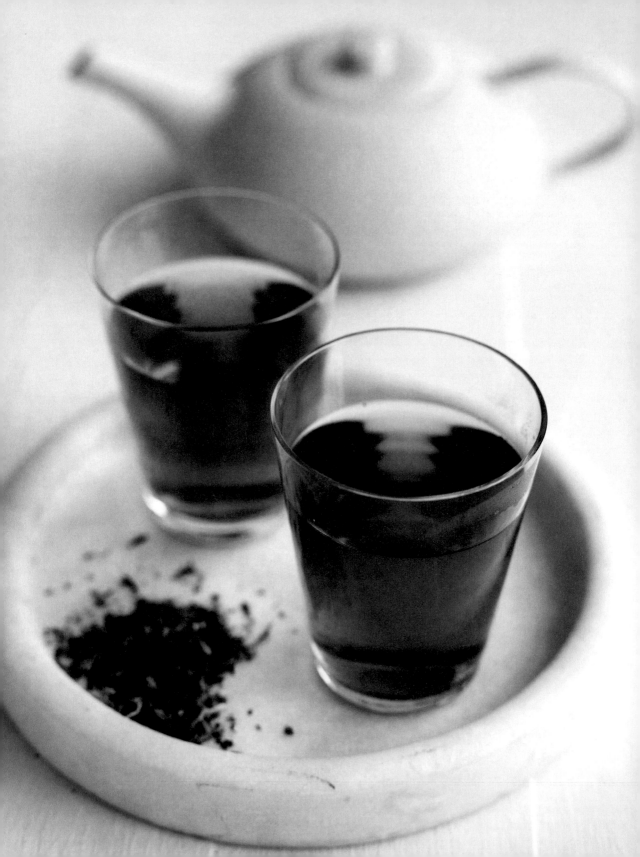

DANDELION TEA

This beautiful tea is a favorite not only for its great taste but also for its medicinal qualities. Dandelion contains calcium, is high in vitamin K, helps the liver, is high in antioxidants, and can help fight skin infections. Enjoy the tea plain or add your favorite milk of choice like macadamia or hemp.

Fill a mug with boiling water.

Stir in the dried dandelion leaves and infuse for 3 minutes. Strain and serve.

Serves: 1

2 tsp dried dandelion tea leaves

NUTRITION INFORMATION

calories 0 | 0g total fat (0g saturated fat, 0g trans fat) | 0mgcholesterol
9.5mg sodium | 0g total carbohydrate (0g dietary fiber, 0g total sugars, -g added sugars)
0g protein | 0mcg vitamin D | 7.1mg calcium | 0mg iron | 0mg potassium

FISH TEA

Fish tea might seem like a really strange idea, but it is actually a light, refreshing beverage and also very nourishing on so many levels. I encourage you to give this quick recipe a try. You'll be pleasantly surprised by the flavor.

Serves: 1

1½ cups Fish Broth (page 172)

1 Tbsp coconut oil or good-quality animal fat

Sea salt

½ tsp lemon juice or apple cider vinegar (optional)

Heat the broth in a saucepan until just simmering. Stir in the oil and season with salt to taste.

Add some lemon juice or vinegar (if using).

Pour the broth into a mug and serve.

NUTRITION INFORMATION

calories 180.6 | 15.7g total fat (11.7g saturated fat, 0g trans fat) | 0mg cholesterol
1309mg sodium | 1.5g total carbohydrate (0g dietary fiber, 0.3g total sugars, -g added sugars)
7.3g protein | 0mcg vitamin D | 110.4mg calcium | 0.8mg iron | 316.6mg potassium

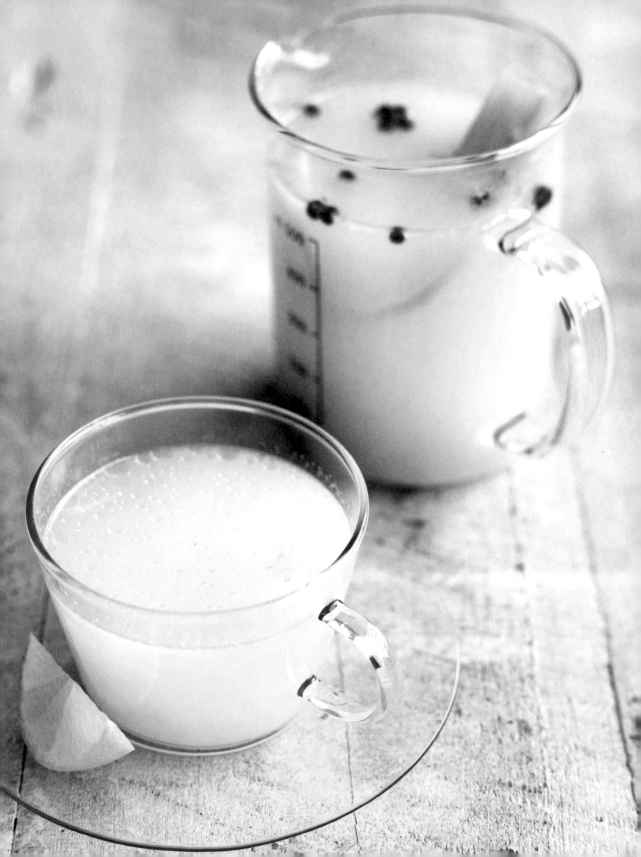

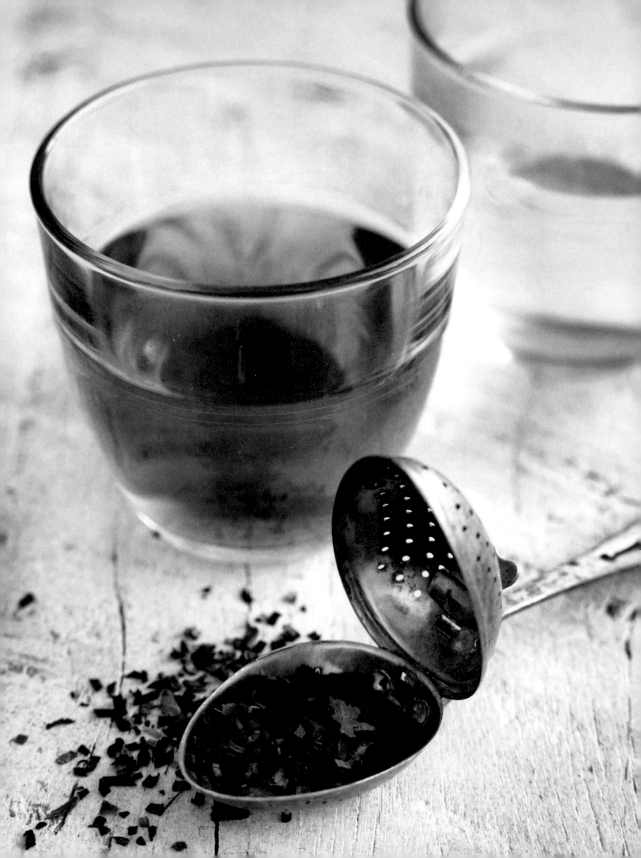

HONEYBUSH TEA

Honeybush tea is a favorite of South Africans along with its cousin plant, rooibos. The leaves come from a shrub with a honey-like scent that gives the plant and this tea its sweet-sounding name. The flavor of the tea is floral, lightly roasted, and similar to honey. Honeybush is known to calm coughs, help with menopausal systems, and decrease blood sugar. If you can't find honeybush, try some rooibos instead.

Fill a mug with boiling water.

Stir in the honeybush tea leaves and allow to infuse for 3 minutes. Strain and serve.

Serves: 1

2 tsp dried honeybush or rooibos tea leaves

NUTRITION INFORMATION
calories 0 | 0g total fat (0g saturated fat, 0g trans fat) | 0mg cholesterol
9.5mg sodium | 0g total carbohydrate (0g dietary fiber, 0g total sugars, -g added sugars)
0g protein | 0mcg vitamin D | 7.1mg calcium | 0mg iron | 0mg potassium

MITOMIX COFFEE/TEA

Dave Asprey from Bulletproof Coffee created a worldwide phenomenon with his approach to coffee by adding in good-quality fat, and of course using the most premium coffee beans. We pay respect to the idea and use the foundational principles behind it to add even more healthy fat, which can help fuel the brain and body.

Serves: 1

1 cup (approximately 8 oz) hot black coffee, strong black tea, or herbal tea of your choice

1 Tbsp coconut oil

1 Tbsp MCT oil or 1 Tbsp organic grass-fed butter

Sweetener (such as stevia, monk fruit [lo han kuo], or xylitol), to taste (optional)

Ground cinnamon, to taste (optional)

Place the coffee, coconut oil, MCT oil, and sweetener of your choice (if using) in a blender and blend for 10 seconds or until the mixture becomes pale in color. Pour into a coffee cup or latte glass, sprinkle a little cinnamon over the top, and serve.

NUTRITION INFORMATION

calories 241.7 | 27.5g total fat (24.5g saturated fat, 0g trans fat) | 0mg cholesterol
7.2mg sodium | 1.2g total carbohydrate (0.3g dietary fiber, 0g total sugars, -g added sugars)
0g protein | 0mcg vitamin D | 6.6mg calcium | 0.1mg iron | 90.5mg potassium

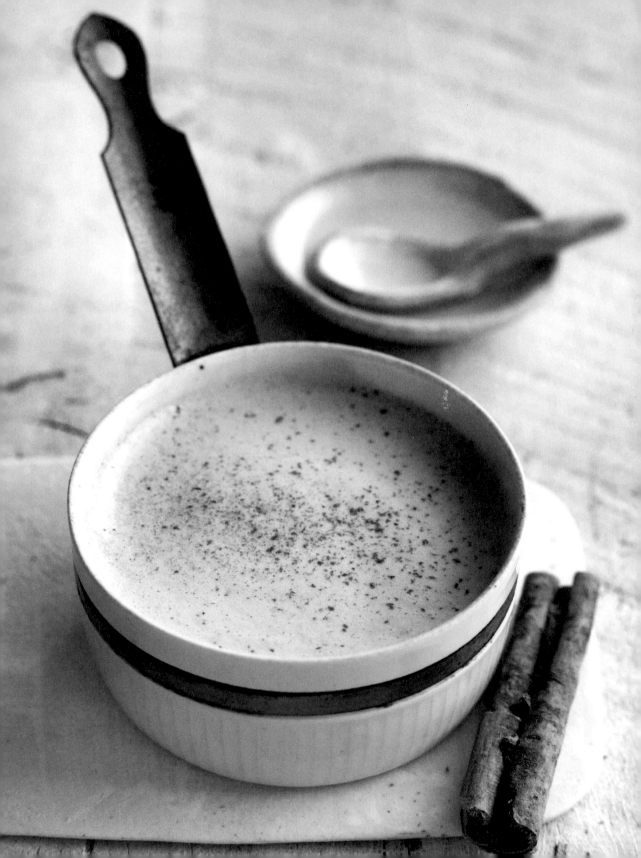

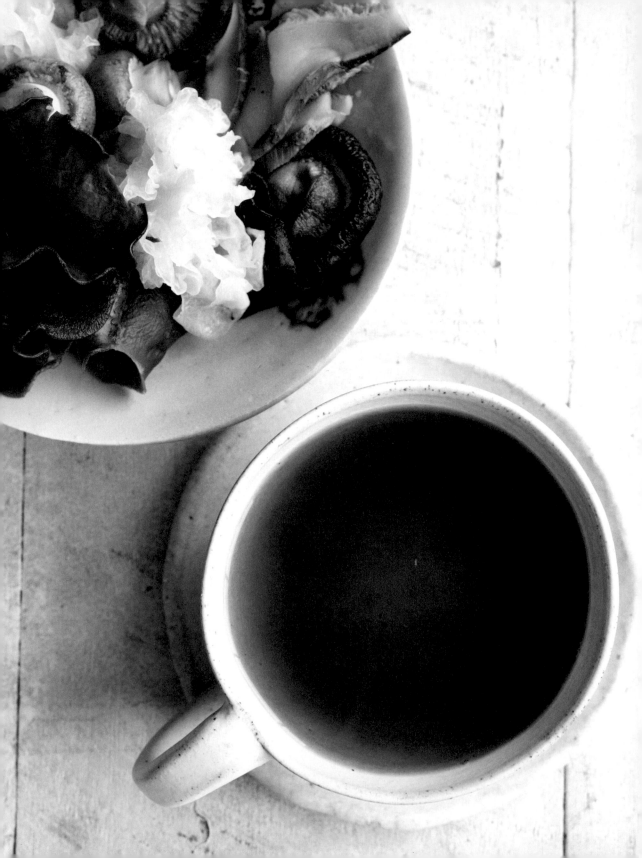

MUSHROOM TEA

Mushrooms are quickly becoming the darling of the health world because of their medicinal properties, and people are now incorporating them into their diets as part of a daily health regimen. A wonderful way to do so in a whole-food form is to simply simmer mushrooms in some good-quality water and let the flavors develop into a delicious tea.

Heat the broth in a saucepan until just simmering. Stir in the oil and season with salt to taste.

Pour the broth into a mug and serve.

Serves: 1

1½ cups Mushroom Broth (page 168)

1 Tbsp coconut oil or good-quality animal fat

Sea salt

NUTRITION INFORMATION

calories 211.6 | 13.7g total fat (11.3g saturated fat, 0g trans fat) | 0mg cholesterol
196.2mg sodium | 21.7g total carbohydrate (6.5g dietary fiber, 1.5g total sugars, -g added sugars)
2.4g protein | 0.6mcg vitamin D | 34mg calcium | 3.4mg iron | 356.6mg potassium

PETE'S SUPER BROTH TEA

Pete has been consuming bone broths on a daily basis for the past 10 years. He decided to take this broth to another level with the added flavor of turmeric, along with ginger, lemon juice, black pepper, and some sea salt. Play with different herbs and spices to see what you like, and feel free to add a clove of chopped garlic along with some MCT oil for richness and to get extra good fats into your body.

Serves: 1

1½ cups Chicken Bone Broth (page 164; you can substitute beef, fish, or pork bone broth)

½ tsp finely grated ginger

½ tsp finely grated turmeric or ¼ tsp ground turmeric

¼ tsp finely grated garlic

½ to 1 tsp lemon juice, or enough to taste

1 Tbsp coconut oil or good-quality animal fat

Sea salt and freshly ground black pepper

Heat the broth in a saucepan until just simmering. Stir in the ginger, turmeric, garlic, lemon juice, and oil. Season with salt and pepper to taste.

Pour the broth into a mug and serve.

NUTRITION INFORMATION

calories 207.6 | 18g total fat (12.6g saturated fat, 0.1g trans fat) | 3.9mg cholesterol
668.1mg sodium | 3.1g total carbohydrate (0.3g dietary fiber, 0.8g total sugars, -g added sugars)
8.2g protein | 0.1mcg vitamin D | 20mg calcium | 1.2mg iron | 348.2mg potassium

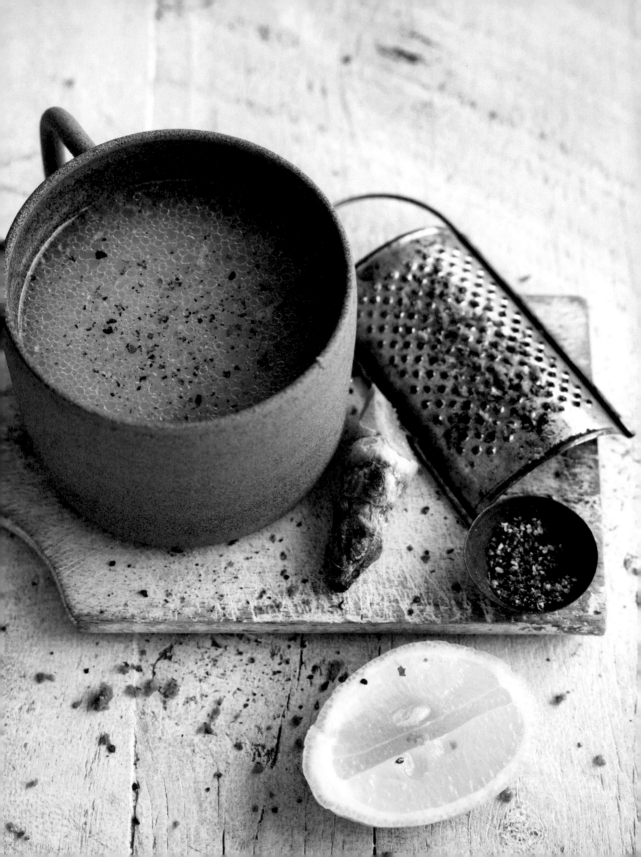

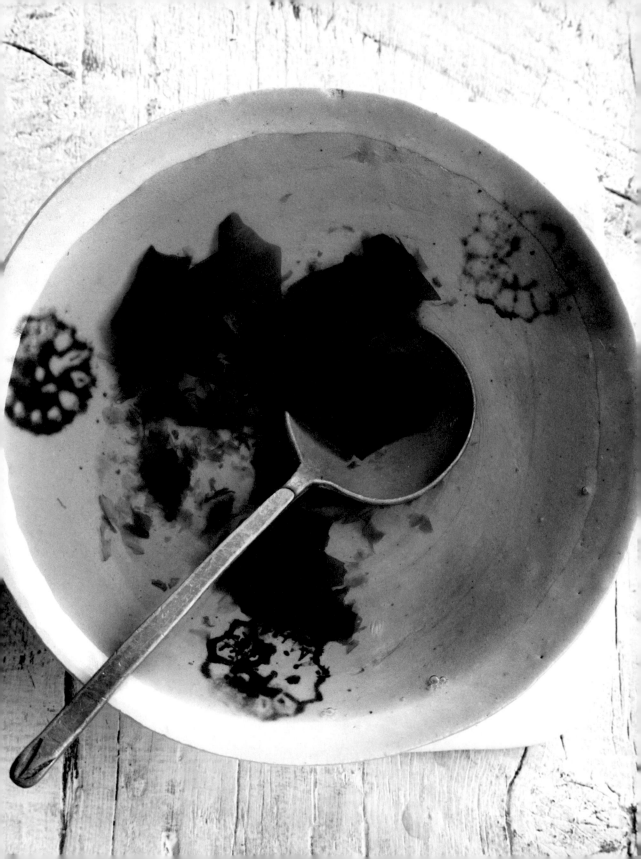

SEAWEED TEA

One of the wonderful ingredients in seaweed and sea vegetables is iodine. For this reason, you should try to eat seaweed a few times a week—plus, it's delicious. Make this wonderful tea to enjoy straight up or to use as a base for tasty soups.

Place the broth in a saucepan. Stir in the wakame.

Place over medium heat, bring to a simmer, then turn down to low and gently simmer for 15 minutes for the seaweed to expand and infuse. Stir in the tamari and oil. Add a little salt to taste.

Pour the broth into a mug and serve.

Serves: 1

1½ cups Fish Broth (page 172) (you can substitute chicken broth)

1 Tbsp dried wakame seaweed

½ tsp tamari or coconut aminos

1 Tbsp coconut oil or good-quality animal fat

Sea salt or more tamari to taste

NUTRITION INFORMATION

calories 257.6 | 15.7g total fat (11.7g saturated fat, 0g trans fat) | 0mg cholesterol
3343.9mg sodium | 14g total carbohydrate (12g dietary fiber, 0.8g total sugars, 0g added sugars)
13.3g protein | 0mcg vitamin D | 350mg calcium | 5.1mg iron | 1754.8mg potassium

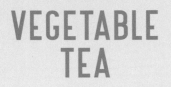

VEGETABLE TEA

One of the first stocks Pete learned to cook as a young chef was a simple vegetable stock. Even though it doesn't have the same flavor profile of chicken or beef broth, it can be very beneficial in cooking as it can be the base for vegetable purees and for poaching vegetables. For anyone who chooses to not eat meat or seafood, vegetable, mushroom, and seaweed broths are great alternatives.

Serves: 1

1½ cups Vegetable Broth (page 172)

1 Tbsp coconut oil or good-quality animal fat

Sea salt

Pinch of ground turmeric (optional)

Heat the broth in a saucepan until just simmering. Stir in the oil. Season with some salt to taste and turmeric, if desired.

Pour the broth into a mug and serve.

NUTRITION INFORMATION

calories 175.6 | 15.1g total fat (12.4g saturated fat, 0g trans fat) | 0mg cholesterol
224.9mg sodium | 9.3g total carbohydrate (2.8g dietary fiber, 3.1g total sugars, -g added sugars)
1.8g protein | 0mcg vitamin D | 50.1mg calcium | 1.3mg iron | 341mg potassium

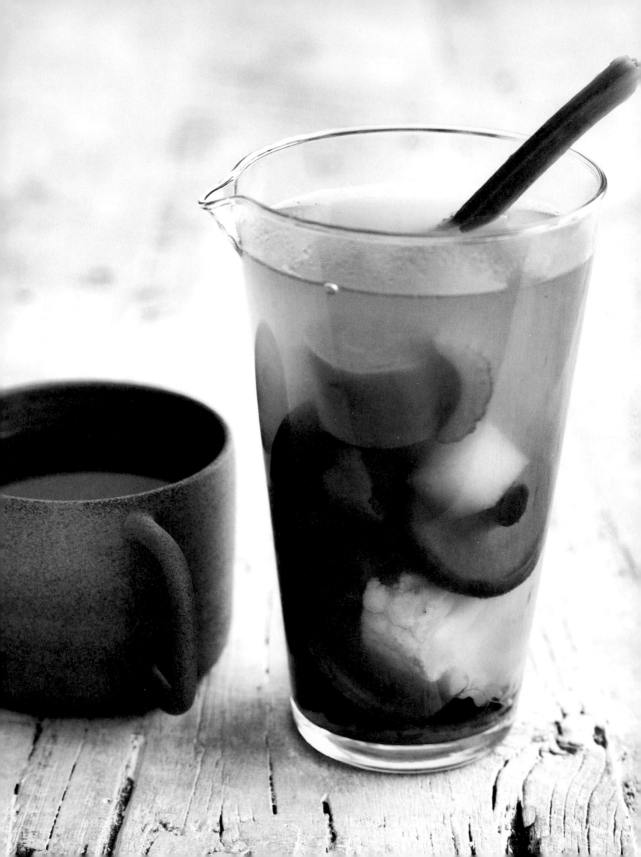

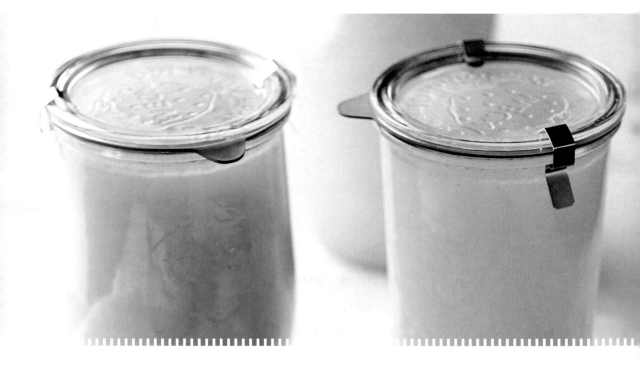

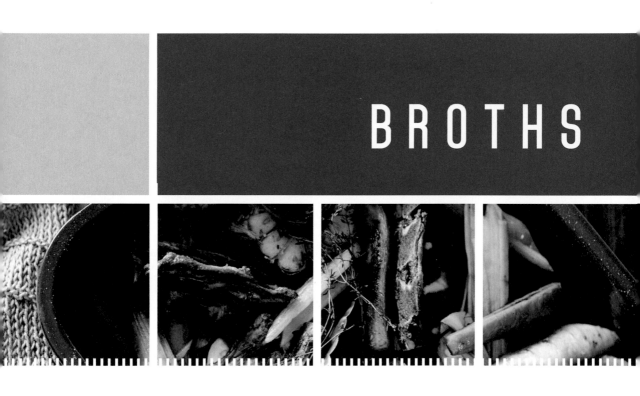

BROTHS

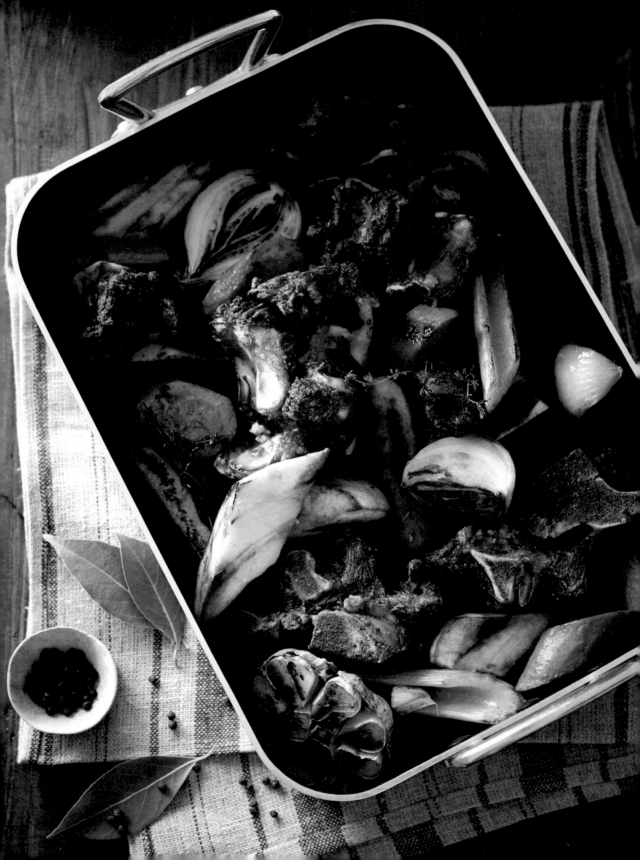

BEEF BONE BROTH

If you have read any of Pete's other cookbooks, you will know by now how important bone broth is for your gut and overall health. Making and storing a big batch of this simple beef broth comes in handy when you want something in the morning to get you through to lunchtime, or when you don't want a full meal at the end of the day.

Place the knuckle and marrowbones in a stockpot. Add the vinegar and pour in 5 quarts of cold filtered water, or enough to cover the bones. Set aside for 1 hour to help draw out the nutrients from the bones. Remove the bones from the pot, reserving the water in a separate container.

Preheat the oven to 350°F.

Place the knuckle and marrowbones, along with the meaty beef bones, in a large roasting pan (if bones are crowded, use multiple roasting pans so that more of their surfaces are exposed to the air and can brown) and roast in the oven for 30 to 40 minutes, until well browned. Return all the bones to the stockpot and add the onions, carrots, celery, and leeks.

Pour the fat from the roasting pan(s) into a saucepan and add 4 cups of water. Place over high heat and bring to a simmer, stirring with a wooden spoon to loosen any coagulated juices. Transfer this liquid to the bones and vegetables in the stockpot. If necessary, add the more water to just cover the bones; the liquid should come no higher than ¾ inch below the rim of the pot, as the volume will increase slightly during cooking.

Bring the broth to a boil, skimming off any scum that rises to the top. Reduce the heat to low and add the thyme, bay leaves, peppercorns, and garlic. Simmer for 12 to 24 hours. Just before finishing, add the parsley and simmer for 10 minutes. Strain the broth into a large container, cover, and place in the fridge overnight.

Remove the congealed fat that rises to the top and reserve for cooking; it will keep in the fridge for up to 1 week or in the freezer for up to 3 months. Transfer the thick and gelatinous broth to smaller airtight containers. The broth can be stored in the fridge for 3 to 4 days or in the freezer for up to 3 months.

Makes: 3½ to 4 quarts

About 4½ lb beef knuckle and marrowbones

3 Tbsp apple cider vinegar

3 lb meaty beef rib or neck bones

3 onions, roughly chopped

3 carrots, roughly chopped

3 celery stalks, roughly chopped

2 leeks (white part only), roughly chopped

3 thyme sprigs

2 bay leaves

1 tsp black peppercorns, crushed

1 garlic bulb, cut in half horizontally

2 large handfuls flat-leaf parsley stalks

NUTRITION INFORMATION

calories 20.6 | 0g total fat (0g saturated fat, 0g trans fat) | 0mg cholesterol
475.7mg sodium | 0.6g total carbohydrate (0g dietary fiber, 0.5g total sugars, -g added sugars)
4.7g protein | 0mcg vitamin D | 14.7mg calcium | 0.8mg iron | 442.8mg potassium

CHICKEN BONE BROTH

Out of all the broths, chicken is the most user-friendly and the one that everyone seems to love the most when it comes to flavor. Chicken broth is also so built into the psyche that it is pure nourishment for when you are sick, so why not have it every day to avoid the sickness?

Makes: 3½ to 4 quarts

2½ lb bony chicken parts (I like to use necks, backs, breastbones, and wings)

2 to 4 chicken feet (optional)

2 Tbsp apple cider vinegar

1 large onion, roughly chopped

2 carrots, roughly chopped

3 celery stalks, roughly chopped

2 leeks (white part only), roughly chopped

1 garlic bulb, cut in half horizontally

1 Tbsp black peppercorns, lightly crushed

2 bay leaves

2 large handfuls flat-leaf parsley stalks

Place the chicken parts in a stockpot. Add 5 quarts of cold filtered water and the remaining ingredients and let stand for 1½ hours to help draw out the nutrients from the bones.

Place the pot over medium-high heat and bring to a boil, skimming off any scum that forms on the surface of the liquid. Reduce the heat to low and simmer for 12 to 24 hours. The longer you cook the broth, the richer and more flavorful it will be.

Strain the broth through a fine sieve into a large storage container, cover, and place in the fridge overnight until the fat rises to the top and congeals. Skim off the fat and reserve for cooking; it will keep in the fridge for up to 1 week or in the freezer for up to 3 months. Transfer the broth to smaller airtight containers. The broth can be stored in the fridge for 3 to 4 days or in the freezer for up to 3 months.

NUTRITION INFORMATION
calories 52.3 | 2.9g total fat (0.9g saturated fat, 0g trans fat) | 2.6mg cholesterol
341.5mg sodium | 0.9g total carbohydrate (0g dietary fiber, 0.4g total sugars, -g added sugars)
5.3g protein | 0.1mcg vitamin D | 10.6mg calcium | 0.5mg iron | 205.7mg potassium

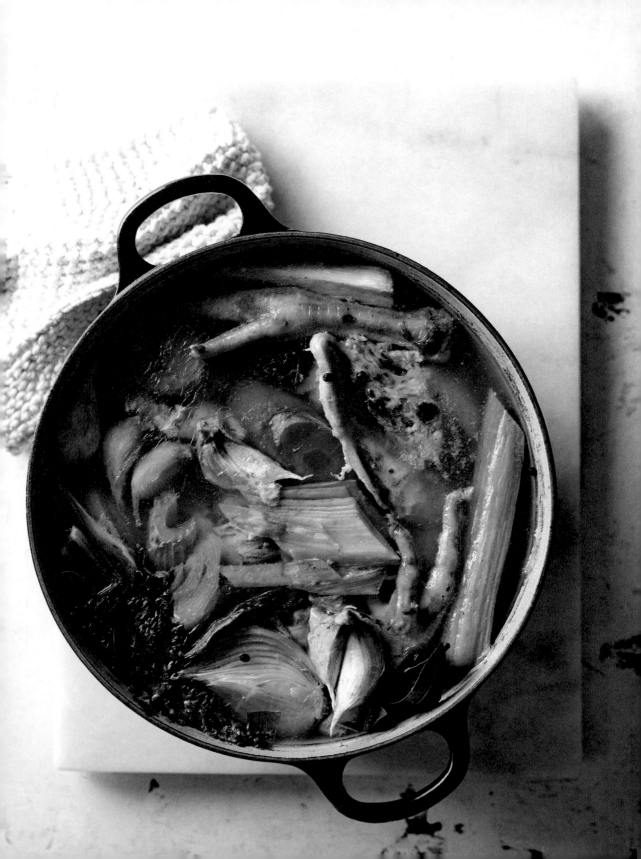

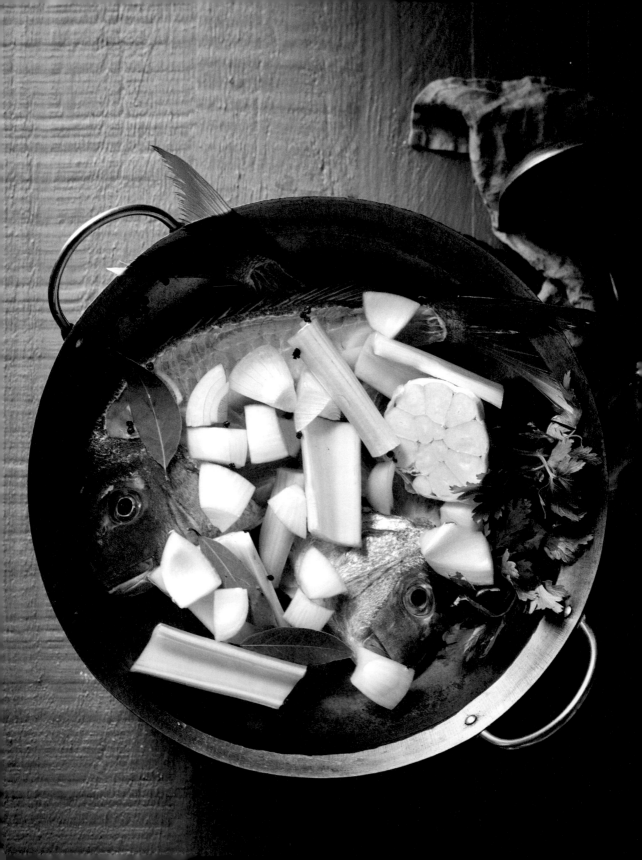

FISH BROTH

This fish broth might seem like a really strange idea to consume straight, but it is actually very delicious and also nourishing on so many levels. Pete's daughters make this broth when they have leftover fish bones from fishing. If drinking straight-up fish broth doesn't appeal to you, then add in some veggies, fish, and spices to turn it into a wonderful seafood soup.

Melt the oil in a stockpot or large saucepan over medium-low heat. Add the vegetables and cook gently for 30 to 60 minutes, until soft. Pour in the wine, if using, and bring to a boil. Add the fish carcasses and cover with 3½ quarts of cold water. Stir in the vinegar and bring to a boil, skimming off the scum and any impurities as they rise to the top.

Tie the herbs together with kitchen string and add to the pot. Reduce the heat to low, cover, and simmer for at least 3 hours. Remove the fish carcasses with tongs or a slotted spoon and strain the liquid through a sieve into a large storage container. Cover and place in the fridge overnight so that the fat rises to the top and congeals.

Remove the fat and reserve it for cooking; it will keep in the fridge for up to 1 week or in the freezer for up to 3 months. Transfer the broth to smaller airtight containers. The broth should be thick and gelatinous—the longer you cook the bones, the more gelatinous it will become. Store in the fridge for 3 to 4 days or in the freezer for up to 3 months.

Makes: 3 quarts

2 Tbsp coconut oil

2 celery stalks, roughly chopped

2 onions, roughly chopped

1 carrot, roughly chopped

½ cup dry white wine (optional)

3 or 4 whole fish carcasses (including heads), such as snapper, barramundi, or kingfish

3 tablespoons apple cider vinegar

1 handful thyme sprigs and flat-leaf parsley

NUTRITION INFORMATION

calories 37.3 | 1.4g total fat (0.3g saturated fat, 0g trans fat) | 0mg cholesterol
363.5mg sodium | 0.9g total carbohydrate (0g dietary fiber, 0.2g total sugars, -g added sugars)
4.7g protein | 0mcg vitamin D | 69.9mg calcium | 0.5mg iron | 200.4mg potassium

MUSHROOM BROTH

There's a good reason to add mushrooms to just about any recipe you can: They're excellent for your health! This broth has a carefully balanced flavor structure that consists of aromatic mushrooms, garlic, and onions. The combination of savory ingredients makes a fragrant, rich broth that can be used in virtually any dish.

Makes: about 2½ quarts

1 cup dried shiitake mushrooms

½ cup dried wood ear mushrooms

1 cup fresh mixed mushrooms and stems of your choice (such as portobello, swiss, button, cup, or shiitake)

3 thyme sprigs

2 bay leaves

1 onion, roughly chopped

1 stalk celery

1 head of garlic, halved

1 tsp peppercorns

Place the dried and fresh mushrooms in a large saucepan. Add 3½ quarts of water and all the remaining ingredients. Place the saucepan over medium-high heat and bring to a boil. Reduce the heat to low, cover with a lid, and simmer for 3 to 4 hours. The longer you cook the broth, the richer and more flavorful it will be.

Strain the broth into a storage container. Store in the fridge for up to 1 week or in the freezer for up to 3 months.

NUTRITION INFORMATION

calories 60.1 | 0.1g total fat (0g saturated fat, 0g trans fat) | 0mg cholesterol
27.4mg sodium | 14.5g total carbohydrate (4.3g dietary fiber, 1g total sugars, -g added sugars)
1.6g protein | 0.4mcg vitamin D | 22.5mg calcium | 2.2mg iron | 237.7mg potassium

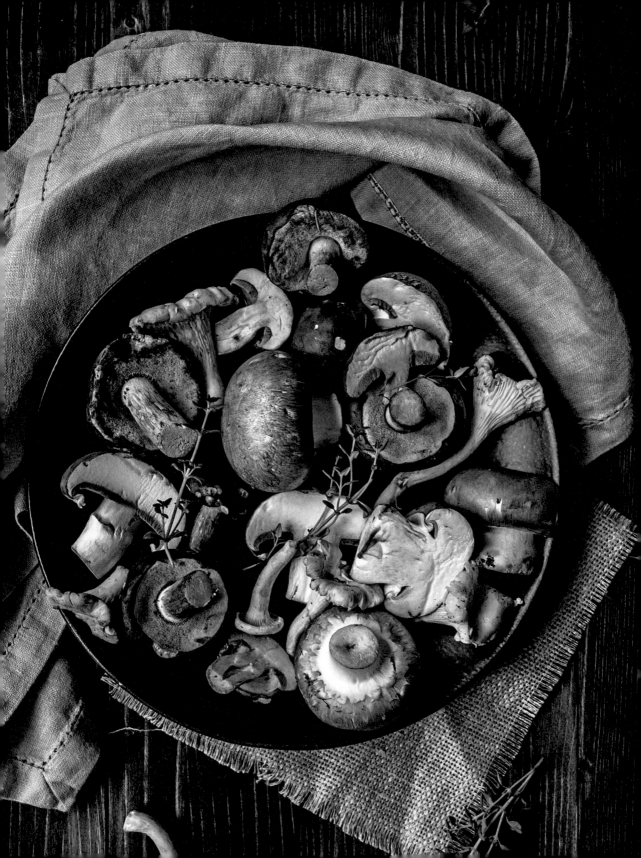

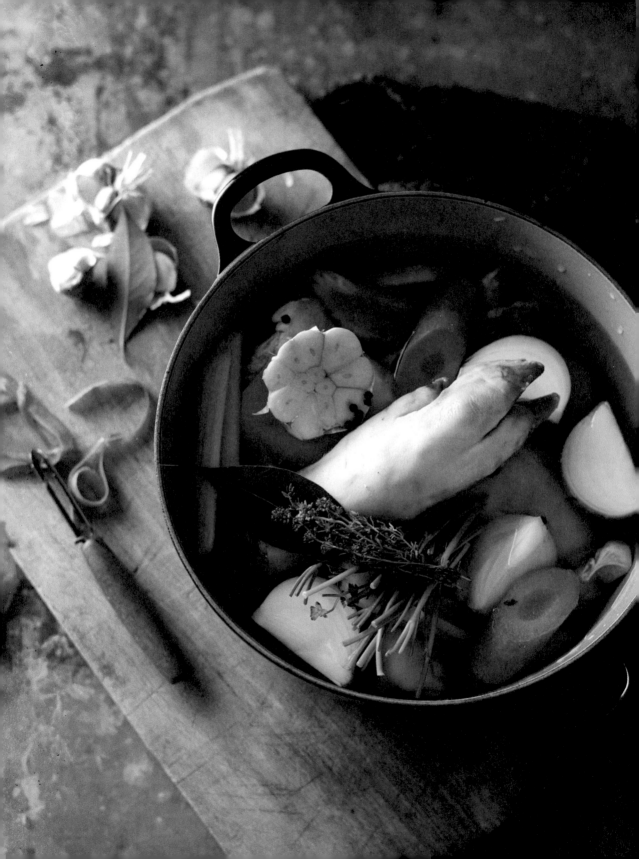

PORK BONE BROTH

Pork bone broth is revered in Japan, China, Vietnam, and many European countries. The reason it has become a part of so many national cuisines is because of the flavor that comes from the simple process of simmering pork bones and water together for hours upon hours. You can flavor this broth with spices or herbs, or add in some meat and vegetables to make a rich and nourishing soup.

Place the pork bones and trotters in a stockpot. Add the vinegar and pour in 5 quarts of cold filtered water, or enough to cover. Set aside for 1 hour to help draw out the nutrients from the bones. Remove the bones from the pot, reserving the water in a separate container.

Preheat the oven to 350°F.

Place the bones and trotters in a large roasting pan and roast in the oven for 30 to 40 minutes, until well browned. Return all the bones and trotters to the stockpot and add the vegetables.

Pour the fat from the roasting pan into a saucepan. Add 1 quart of the reserved water, place over high heat, and bring to a simmer, stirring with a wooden spoon to loosen any coagulated juices. Add this liquid to the bones and vegetables. If necessary, add the remaining reserved water to the pot to just cover the bones—the liquid should come no higher than ¾ inch below the rim of the pot, as the volume will increase slightly during cooking.

Bring the broth to a boil, skimming off any scum that rises to the top. Reduce the heat to low and add the thyme, bay leaves, peppercorns, and garlic. Simmer for 12 to 24 hours. Just before finishing, add the parsley and simmer for 10 minutes. Strain the broth into a large container, cover, and place in the fridge overnight.

Remove the congealed fat that rises to the top and reserve for cooking; it will keep in the fridge for up to 1 week or in the freezer for up to 3 months. Transfer the broth to smaller airtight containers. The broth can be stored in the fridge for 3 to 4 days or in the freezer for up to 3 months.

Makes: 3½ to 4 quarts

About 8 lb pork bones and trotters

3 Tbsp apple cider vinegar

3 onions, roughly chopped

3 carrots, roughly chopped

3 celery stalks, roughly chopped

2 leeks (white part only), roughly chopped

3 thyme sprigs

2 bay leaves

1 tsp black peppercorns, crushed

1 garlic bulb, cut in half horizontally

2 large handfuls flat-leaf parsley stalks

NUTRITION INFORMATION

calories 13.2 | 0g total fat (0g saturated fat, 0g trans fat) | 0mg cholesterol
480mg sodium | 0.4g total carbohydrate (0g dietary fiber, 0.3g total sugars, -g added sugars)
3g protein | 0mcg vitamin D | 10.8mg calcium | 0.5mg iron | 150mg potassium

VEGETABLE BROTH

The great thing about broth is that it's completely versatile, so you can incorporate a variety of flavors to your liking. Aside from providing different flavors, all the vegetables in this dish have their own set of nutritional components that may help improve your immune function.

Makes: about 3½ quarts

1 Tbsp coconut oil

1 onion, roughly chopped

2 large carrots, roughly chopped

2 parsnips, roughly chopped

1 celery stalk, roughly chopped

¼ head cauliflower, broken into florets (about 8 ounces)

¼ bunch spinach (about 3 ounces)

1 cup mushrooms (portobello, swiss, button, cup, or shiitake, or any mushrooms of your choice)

Several thyme sprigs

Several flat-leaf parsley stalks

1 dried bay leaf

Melt the oil over medium-high heat in a stockpot or large saucepan. Add the onion and cook, stirring, for about 3 minutes, or until translucent. Add the carrot, parsnip, celery, and cauliflower and cook for about 10 minutes, or until slightly tender.

Wash and drain the spinach thoroughly and chop into 1½-inch pieces. Add to the pot, along with 4 quarts of water and the mushrooms, thyme, parsley, and bay leaf. Bring to a boil. Reduce the heat to low, cover, and simmer for about 3 to 4 hours, or until the broth is highly flavored.

Remove the stock from the heat and strain through a fine sieve, pressing on the vegetables to extract all their juices. Pour into storage containers for the fridge or freezer. Discard the vegetables, unless you are keeping them to use in soups.

The broth can be refrigerated for 3 to 4 days or frozen for up to 3 months.

NUTRITION INFORMATION

calories 34.4 | 1.1g total fat (0.8g saturated fat, 0g trans fat) | 0mg cholesterol
53.2mg sodium | 5.8g total carbohydrate (1.7g dietary fiber, 2.1g total sugars, -g added sugars)
1.1g protein | 0mcg vitamin D | 32.2mg calcium | 0.6mg iron | 216.5mg potassium

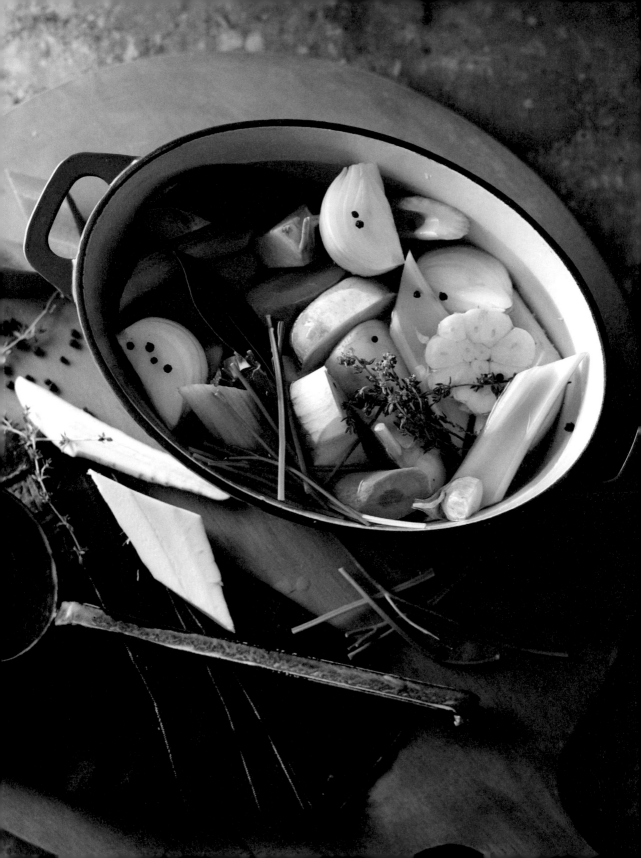

METRIC CONVERSION CHART

The recipes in this book use the standard United States method for measuring liquid and dry or solid ingredients (teaspoons, tablespoons, and cups). The following charts are provided to help cooks outside the U.S. successfully use these recipes. All equivalents are approximate.

Standard Cup	Fine Powder (e.g., flour)	Grain (e.g., rice)	Granular (e.g., sugar)	Liquid Solids (e.g., butter)	Liquid (e.g., milk)
1	140 g	150 g	190 g	200 g	240 ml
¾	105 g	113 g	143 g	150 g	180 ml
⅔	93 g	100 g	125 g	133 g	160 ml
½	70 g	75 g	95 g	100 g	120 ml
⅓	47 g	50 g	63 g	67 g	80 ml
¼	35 g	38 g	48 g	50 g	60 ml
⅛	18 g	19 g	24 g	25 g	30 ml

Useful Equivalents for Liquid Ingredients by Volume					
¼ tsp				1 ml	
½ tsp				2 ml	
1 tsp				5 ml	
3 tsp	1 tbsp		½ fl oz	15 ml	
	2 tbsp	⅛ cup	1 fl oz	30 ml	
	4 tbsp	¼ cup	2 fl oz	60 ml	
	5⅓ tbsp	⅓ cup	3 fl oz	80 ml	
	8 tbsp	½ cup	4 fl oz	120 ml	
	10⅔ tbsp	⅔ cup	5 fl oz	160 ml	
	12 tbsp	¾ cup	6 fl oz	180 ml	
	16 tbsp	1 cup	8 fl oz	240 ml	
	1 pt	2 cups	16 fl oz	480 ml	
	1 qt	4 cups	32 fl oz	960 ml	
			33 fl oz	1000 ml	1 L

Useful Equivalents for Dry Ingredients by Weight		
(To convert ounces to grams, multiply the number of ounces by 30.)		
1 oz	1/16 lb	30 g
4 oz	1/4 lb	120 g
8 oz	1/2 lb	240 g
12 oz	3/4 lb	360 g
16 oz	1 lb	480 g

Useful Equivalents for Cooking/Oven Temperatures			
Process	Fahrenheit	Celsius	Gas Mark
Freeze Water	32° F	0° C	
Room Temperature	68° F	20° C	
Boil Water	212° F	100° C	
Bake	325° F	160° C	3
	350° F	180° C	4
	375° F	190° C	5
	400° F	200° C	6
	425° F	220° C	7
	450° F	230° C	8
Broil			Grill

Useful Equivalents for Length				
(To convert inches to centimeters, multiply the number of inches by 2.5.)				
1 in			2.5 cm	
6 in	1/2 ft		15 cm	
12 in	1 ft		30 cm	
36 in	3 ft	1 yd	90 cm	
40 in			100 cm	1 m

ENDNOTES

Introduction to Fasting

1. M. La Merrill et al., "Toxicological Function of Adipose Tissue: Focus on Persistent Organic Pollutants," *Environmental Health Perspectives* 121, no. 2 (2013): 162–169. DOI: 10.1289 /ehp.1205485. https://www.ncbi.nlm.nih.gov/pmc/articles/PMC3569688/.

2. O. Hue et al., "Increased Plasma Levels of Toxic Pollutants Accompanying Weight Loss Induced by Hypocaloric Diet or by Bariatric Surgery," *Obesity Surgery* 16, no. 9 (2006): 1145– 54. DOI: 10.1381/096089206778392356. https://www.ncbi.nlm.nih.gov/pubmed/16989697.

3. M. J. Kim et al., "Fate and Complex Pathogenic Effects of Dioxins and Polychlorinated Biphenyls in Obese Subjects before and after Drastic Weight Loss," *Environmental Health Perspectives* 119, no. 3 (2011): 377–383. DOI: 10.1289/ehp.1002848.

4. Ibid.

Is Fasting Safe?

1. M. La Merrill et al., "Toxicological Function of Adipose Tissue: Focus on Persistent Organic Pollutants," *Environmental Health Perspectives* 121, no. 2 (2013). 162–169. DOI: 10.1289 /ehp.1205485. https://www.ncbi.nlm.nih.gov/pmc/articles/PMC3569688/.

2. Y. Y. Qin et al., "Persistent Organic Pollutants and Heavy Metals in Adipose Tissues of Patients with Uterine Leiomyomas and the Association of These Pollutants with Seafood Diet, BMI, and Age," *Environmental Science and Pollution Research* 17, no. 1 (2010): 229–240. DOI: 10.1007 /s11356-009-0251-0. https://link.springer.com/article/10.1007%2Fs11356-009-0251-0.

Food and Drink for Keto Fasting

1. L. Gamet-Payrastre et al., "Sulforaphane, a Naturally Occurring Isothiocyanate, Induces Cell Cycle Arrest and Apoptosis in HT29 Human Colon Cancer Cells," *Cancer Research* 60, no. 5 (2000): 1426–33. https://www.ncbi.nlm.nih.gov/pubmed/10728709.

2. A. Wiczk et al., "Sulforaphane, a Cruciferous Vegetable-Derived Isothiocyanate, Inhibits Protein Synthesis in Human Prostate Cancer Cells," *BBA Molecular Cell Research* 1823, no. 8 (2012): 1295–1305. DOI: 10.1016/j.bbamcr.2012.05.020. https://www.sciencedirect.com/science /article/pii/S016748891200136X.

3. Y. Li et al., "Sulforaphane, a Dietary Component of Broccoli/Broccoli Sprouts, Inhibits Breast Cancer Stem Cells," *Clinical Cancer Research* 16, no. 9 (2010): 2580–2590. DOI: 10.1158/1078 -0432.CCR-09-2937.

4. C. C. Conaway et al., "Phenethyl Isothiocyanate and Sulforaphane and Their N-acetylcysteine Conjugates Inhibit Malignant Progression of Lung Adenomas Induced by Tobacco Carcinogens in A/J Mice," *Cancer Research* 65, no. 18 (2005): 8548–57. DOI: 10.1158/0008-5472.CAN-05 -0237. https://www.ncbi.nlm.nih.gov/pubmed/16166336.

5. *M. F. Ullah*, "Sulforaphane (SFN): An Isothiocyanate in a Cancer Chemoprevention Paradigm," *Medicines* 2, no. 3 (2015): 141–156, DOI: 10.3390/medicines2030141. https://www.mdpi .com/2305-6320/2/3/141.

6. E. Munters et al., "Effects of Broccoli Sprouts Intake on Oxidative Stress, Inflammation, Microalbuminuria and Platelet Function in Human Volunteers: a Cross-Over Study," *Proceedings of The Nutrition Society* 69, no. OE68 (2010): E590. DOI: 10.1017 /S0029665110004842. https://www.cambridge.org/core/journals/proceedings-of-the -nutrition-society/article/effects-of-broccoli-sprouts-intake-on-oxidative-stress-inflammation -microalbuminuria-and-platelet-function-in-human-volunteers-a-crossover-study /0DEDA73F445B67B4E3DCDB7B415A48DA.

7. J. Caba, "Eat Your Broccoli: Phenolic Compounds Found in Cruciferous Vegetables Are About to Get a Lot Healthier," Medical Daily June 24, 2016, https://www.medicaldaily.com/broccoli -health-benefits-cruciferous-vegetables-390467.

8. University of Illinois at Urbana-Champaign, "More Reasons to Eat Your Broccoli," June 22, 2016, https://phys.org/news/2016-06-broccoli.html.

9. A. M. Gardner, A. F. Brown, and J. A. Juvik, "QTL Analysis for the Identification of Candidate Genes Controlling Phenolic Compound Accumulation in Broccoli (*Brassica oleracea* L. var. *italica*)," *Molecular Breeding* 36, no. 6 (2016): 81. DOI: 10.1007/s11032-016-0497-4. https://link.springer.com/article/10.1007%2Fs11032-016-0497-4.

10. K. M. Dalessandri et al., "Pilot Study: Effect of 3,3'-Diindolylmethane Supplements on Urinary Hormone Metabolites in Postmenopausal Women with a History of Early-Stage Breast Cancer," *Nutrition and Cancer* 50, no. 2 (2004): 161–7. DOI: 10.1207/s15327914nc5002_5. https://www .ncbi.nlm.nih.gov/pubmed/15623462.

11. W. W. Zhang, Z. Feng, and S. A. Narod, "Multiple Therapeutic and Preventive Effects of 3,3'-Diindolylmethane on Cancers Including Prostate Cancer and High Grade Prostatic Intraepithelial Neoplasia," *Journal of Biomedical Research* 28, no. 5 (2014): 339–348. DOI: 10.7555/JBR.28.20140008.

12. J. Wilcox, "Benefits of Broccoli," *Forbes* July 1, 2012, https://www.forbes.com/sites /juliewilcox/2012/07/01/health-benefits-of-broccoli/#2085c7f942e1.

13. M. Xue et al., "Activation of NF-E2-Related Factor-2 Reverses Biochemical Dysfunction of Endothelial Cells Induced by Hyperglycemia Linked to Vascular Disease," *Diabetes* 57, no. 10 (2008): 2809–2817. DOI: doi.org/10.2337/db06-1003.m http://diabetes.diabetesjournals.org /content/early/2008/08/04/db06-1003?maxtoshow=&HITS=10&hits=10&RESULTFORMAT= &author1=Paul+Thornalley&andorexactfulltext=and&searchid=1&FIRSTINDEX=0&sortspec =relevance&resourcetype=HWCIT.

14. BMJ, "High Dietary Fiber Intake Linked to Health Promoting Short Chain Fatty Acids," ScienceDaily September 29, 2015, https://www.sciencedaily.com /releases/2015/09/150929070122.htm.

15. G. V. Senanayake et al., "The Dietary Phase 2 Protein Inducer Sulforaphane Can Normalize the Kidney Epigenome and Improve Blood Pressure in Hypertensive Rats," *American Journal of Hypertension* 25, no. 2 (2012): 229–35. DOI: 10.1038/ajh.2011.200. https://www.ncbi.nlm.nih .gov/pubmed/22052072.

16. R. K. Davidson et al., "Sulforaphane Represses Matrix-Degrading Proteases and Protects Cartilage from Destruction In Vitro and In Vivo," *Arthritis & Rheumatism* 65, no. 12 (2013): 3130–3140. DOI: 10.1002/art.38133.

17. BBC News, "Broccoli: Researchers Say It Slows Arthritis," August 28, 2013, https://www.bbc .com/news/av/health-23863175/broccoli-researchers-say-it-slows-arthritis.

18. A. S. Axelsson et al., "Sulforaphane Reduces Hepatic Glucose Production and Improves Glucose Control in Patients with Type 2 Diabetes," *Science Translational Medicine* 9, no. 394 (2017). DOI: 10.1126/scitranslmed.aah4477. http://stm.sciencemag.org/content /9/394/eaah4477.

19. M. Xue et al., "Activation of NF-E2–Related Factor-2 Reverses Biochemical Dysfunction of Endothelial Cells Induced by Hyperglycemia Linked to Vascular Disease," *Diabetes* 57, no. 10 (2008): 2809–2817. DOI: 10.2337/db06-1003.

20. G. V. Senanayake et al., "The Dietary Phase 2 Protein Inducer Sulforaphane Can Normalize the Kidney Epigenome and Improve Blood Pressure in Hypertensive Rats," *American Journal of Hypertension* 25, no. 2 (2012): 229–35. DOI: 10.1038/ajh.2011.200. https://www.ncbi.nlm.nih .gov/pubmed/22052072.

21. T. Phillips, "The Role of Methylation in Gene Expression," *Nature Education* 1, no. 1 (2008): 116, https://www.nature.com/scitable/topicpage/the-role-of-methylation-in-gene -expression-1070.

22. G. V. Senanayake et al., "The Dietary Phase 2 Protein Inducer Sulforaphane Can Normalize the Kidney Epigenome and Improve Blood Pressure in Hypertensive Rats," *American Journal of Hypertension* 25, no. 2 (2012): 229–35. DOI: 10.1038/ajh.2011.200. https://www.ncbi.nlm.nih .gov/pubmed/22052072.

23. Holistic Health, "H. Pylori: Another Piece to the Puzzle – Part 1," https://player.vimeo.com /video/26847817.

24. M. A. Riedl, A. Saxon, and D. Diaz-Sanchez, "Oral Sulforaphane Increases Phase II Antioxidant Enzymes in the Human Upper Airway," *Clinical Immunology* 130, no. 3 (2009): 244–251. DOI: 10.1016/j.clim.2008.10.007.

25. T. D. Hubbard et al., "Dietary Broccoli Impacts Microbial Community Structure and Attenuates Chemically Induced Colitis in Mice in an Ah Receptor Dependent Manner," *Journal of Functional Foods* 37 (October 2017): 685-698. DOI: 10.1016/j.jff.2017.08.038. https://www .sciencedirect.com/science/article/pii/S1756464617305029.

26. "Broccoli May Ward Off Leaky Gut Problems," *The National* October 15, 2017, https://www .thenational.ae/lifestyle/food/broccoli-may-ward-off-leaky-gut-problems-1.667203.

27. Pennsylvania State University, "Like It or Not: Broccoli May Be Good for the Gut," ScienceDaily October 12, 2017, https://www.sciencedaily.com/releases/2017/10/171012151754.htm.

28. "Broccoli Compounds Could Aid Leaky Gut," Natural Health News October 16, 2017, https://www.naturalhealthnews.uk/food/2017/10/broccoli-compounds-could-aid-leaky-gut/.

29. A. Tarozzi et al., "Sulforaphane as a Potential Protective Phytochemical against Neurodegenerative Diseases," *Oxidative Medicine and Cellular Longevity* (2013): 415078. DOI: 10.1155/2013/415078.

30. L. C. Blekkenhorst et al., "Cruciferous and Total Vegetable Intakes Are Inversely Associated with Subclinical Atherosclerosis in Older Adult Women," *JAHA: Journal of the American Heart Association* 7, no. 8 (2018). DOI: 10.1161/JAHA.117.008391. https://www.ahajournals.org /doi/10.1161/JAHA.117.008391.

31. K. F. Mills et al., "Long-Term Administration of Nicotinamide Mononucleotide Mitigates Age-Associated Physiological Decline in Mice," Cell Metabolism 24, no. 6 (2016): 795–806. DOI: 10.1016/j.cmet.2016.09.013. https://www.sciencedirect.com/science/article/pii /S1550413116304958.

32. Fox News, "Compound in Broccoli May Slow Signs of Aging," October 28, 2016, https://www .foxnews.com/health/compound-in-broccoli-may-slow-signs-of-aging.

33. L. Rusu, "Natural Compound Derived from Broccoli, Avocado Shows Promise in Reducing Signs of Aging," Tech Times October 29, 2016, https://www.techtimes.com/articles /184088/20161029/natural-compound-derived-from-broccoli-avocado-shows-promise-in -reducing-signs-of-aging.htm.

34. C. C. Alano, W. Ying, and R. A. Swanson, "Poly(ADP-ribose) Polymerase-1-mediated Cell Death in Astrocytes Requires NAD+ Depletion and Mitochondrial Permeability Transition," *Journal of Biological Chemistry* 279, no. 18 (2004): 18895–902. DOI: 10.1074/jbc.M313329200. https://www.ncbi.nlm.nih.gov/pubmed/14960594.

35. J. B. Kirkland and M. L. Meyer-Ficca, "Chapter Three – Niacin," *Advances in Food and Nutrition Research* 83 (2018): 83–149. DOI: 10.1016/bs.afnr.2017.11.003. https://www.sciencedirect.com/science/article/pii/S1043452617300396.

36. K. L. Stromsdorfer et al., "NAMPT-Mediated NAD+ Biosynthesis in Adipocytes Regulates Adipose Tissue Function and Multi-organ Insulin Sensitivity in Mice," *Cell Reports* 16, no. 7 (2016): 1851–1860. DOI: 10.1016/j.celrep.2016.07.027. https://www.cell.com/cell-reports /fulltext/S2211-1247(16)30945-7.

37. K. M. Dalessandri et al., "Pilot Study: Effect of 3,3'-Diindolylmethane Supplements on Urinary Hormone Metabolites in Postmenopausal Women with a History of Early-Stage Breast Cancer," *Nutrition and Cancer* 50, no. 2 (2004): 161–7. DOI: 10.1207/s15327914nc5002_5. https://www.ncbi.nlm.nih.gov/pubmed/15623462.

38. W.W. Zhang, Z. Feng, and S.A. Narod, "Multiple Therapeutic and Preventive Effects of 3,3'-Diindolylmethane on Cancers Including Prostate Cancer and High Grade Prostatic Intraepithelial Neoplasia," *Journal of Biomedical Research* 28, no. 5 (2014): 339–348. DOI: 10.7555/JBR.28.20140008. https://www.ncbi.nlm.nih.gov/pmc/articles/PMC4197384/.

39. R. Naik et al., "A Randomized Phase II Trial of Indole-3-Carbinol in the Treatment of Vulvar Intraepithelial Neoplasia," *International Journal of Gynecological Cancer* 16, no. 2 (2006): 786–90. DOI: 10.1111/j.1525-1438.2006.00386.x. https://www.ncbi.nlm.nih.gov/pubmed /16681761.

40. L. Gamet-Payrastre et al., "Sulforaphane, a Naturally Occurring Isothiocyanate, Induces Cell Cycle Arrest and Apoptosis in HT29 Human Colon Cancer Cells," *Cancer Research* 60, no. 5 (2000): 1426–33. https://www.ncbi.nlm.nih.gov/pubmed/10728709.

41. W.W. Zhang, Z. Feng, and S.A. Narod, "Multiple Therapeutic and Preventive Effects of 3,3'-Diindolylmethane on Cancers Including Prostate Cancer and High Grade Prostatic Intraepithelial Neoplasia," *Journal of Biomedical Research* 28, no. 5 (2014): 339–348. DOI: 10.7555/JBR.28.20140008. https://www.ncbi.nlm.nih.gov/pmc/articles/PMC4197384/.

42. A. Wiczk et al., "Sulforaphane, a Cruciferous Vegetable-Derived Isothiocyanate, Inhibits Protein Synthesis in Human Prostate Cancer Cells," *BBA Molecular Cell Research* 1823, no. 8 (2012): 1295–1305. DOI: 10.1016/j.bbamcr.2012.05.020. https://www.sciencedirect.com/science/article/pii/S016748891200136X.

43. Y. Li et al., "Sulforaphane, a Dietary Component of Broccoli/Broccoli Sprouts, Inhibits Breast Cancer Stem Cells," *Clinical Cancer Research* 16, no. 9 (2010): 2580–2590. DOI: 10.1158/1078-0432.CCR-09-2937.

44. C. C. Conaway et al., "Phenethyl Isothiocyanate and Sulforaphane and Their N-acetylcysteine Conjugates Inhibit Malignant Progression of Lung Adenomas Induced by Tobacco Carcinogens in A/J Mice," *Cancer Research* 65, no. 18 (2005): 8548–57. DOI: 10.1158/0008-5472.CAN-05-0237. https://www.ncbi.nlm.nih.gov/pubmed/16166336.

45. S. M. Tortorella et al., "Dietary Sulforaphane in Cancer Chemoprevention: The Role of Epigenetic Regulation and HDAC Inhibition," *Antioxidants & Redox Signaling* 22, no. 16 (2015): 1382–1424. DOI: 10.1089/ars.2014.6097. https://www.ncbi.nlm.nih.gov/pmc/articles/PMC4432495/.

46. A. S. Axelsson et al., "Sulforaphane Reduces Hepatic Glucose Production and Improves Glucose Control in Patients with Type 2 Diabetes," *Science Translational Medicine* 9, no. 394 (2017). DOI: 10.1126/scitranslmed.aah4477. http://stm.sciencemag.org/content/9/394/eaah4477.

47. "British Scientists Have Developed Broccoli Pill to Help in Arthritis Fight," *Daily Express*, April 27, 2015, https://www.express.co.uk/life-style/health/573089/Broccoli-pill-help-arthritis-fight.

48. Y. Li et al., "Sulforaphane, a Dietary Component of Broccoli/Broccoli Sprouts, Inhibits Breast Cancer Stem Cells," *Clinical Cancer Research* 16, no. 9 (2010): 2580–2590. DOI: 10.1158/1078-0432.CCR-09-2937. https://www.ncbi.nlm.nih.gov/pubmed/20388854.

49. S. Lee et al., "Sulforaphane Upregulates the Heat Shock Protein Co-Chaperone CHIP and Clears Amyloid-β and Tau in a Mouse Model of Alzheimer's Disease," *Molecular Nutrition & Food Research* 62, no. 12 (2018): 1800240. DOI: 10.1002/mnfr.201800240. https://www.ncbi.nlm.nih.gov/pubmed/29714053.

50. A. S. Axelsson et al., "Sulforaphane Reduces Hepatic Glucose Production and Improves Glucose Control in Patients with Type 2 Diabetes," *Science Translational Medicine* 9, no. 394 (2017). DOI: 10.1126/scitranslmed.aah4477. http://stm.sciencemag.org/content/9/394/eaah4477.

51. Kanazawa University, "Sulforaphane, a Phytochemical in Broccoli Sprouts, Ameliorates Obesity," *ScienceDaily*, March 7, 2017, https://www.sciencedaily.com/releases/2017/03/170307100402.htm.

52. P. A. Egner et al., "Rapid and Sustainable Detoxication of Airborne Pollutants by Broccoli Sprout Beverage: Results of a Randomized Clinical Trial in China," *Cancer Prevention Research* 7, no. 8 (2014): 813–823. DOI: 10.1158/1940-6207.CAPR-14-0103. https://www.ncbi.nlm.nih.gov/pmc/articles/PMC4125483/.

53. M. Xue et al., "Activation of NF-E2–Related Factor-2 Reverses Biochemical Dysfunction of Endothelial Cells Induced by Hyperglycemia Linked to Vascular Disease," *Diabetes* 57, no. 10 (2008): 2809–2817. DOI: 10.2337/db06-1003. http://diabetes.diabetesjournals.org/content/early/2008/08/04/db06-1003?maxtoshow=&HITS=10&hits=10&RESULTFORMAT=&author1=Paul+Thornalley&andorexactfulltext=and&searchid=1&FIRSTINDEX=0&sortspec=relevance&resourcetype=HWCIT.

54. G. S. Shehatou and G. M. Suddek, "Sulforaphane Attenuates the Development of Atherosclerosis and Improves Endothelial Dysfunction in Hypercholesterolemic Rabbits," *Experimental Biology and Medicine* 241, no. 4 (2016): 426–436. DOI: 10.1177/1535370215609695. https://www.ncbi.nlm.nih.gov/pmc/articles/PMC4935417/.

55. L. M. Beaver et al., "Long Non-Coding RNAs and Sulforaphane: A Target for Chemoprevention and Suppression of Prostate Cancer," *Journal of Nutritional Biochemistry* 42 (2017): 72–83. DOI: 10.1016/j.jnutbio.2017.01.001. https://www.ncbi.nlm.nih.gov/pubmed/28131897.

56. University of Illinois at Urbana-Champaign, "Maximizing the Anti-Cancer Power of Broccoli," *ScienceDaily*, April 5, 2005, https://www.sciencedaily.com/releases/2005/03/050326114810.htm.

57. American Institute for Cancer Research, "New Research Reveals How to Prepare Foods to Boost Cancer-Fighting Activity," November 7, 2013, http://www.aicr.org/press/press-releases/good-food-prep-boosts-cancer-fighting-ability.html?referrer=https://www.google.com/.

58. J. L. Marnewick et al., "Ex Vivo Modulation of Chemical-Induced Mutagenesis by Subcellular Liver Fractions of Rats Treated with Rooibos (*Aspalathus linearis*) Tea, Honeybush (*Cyclopia intermedia*) Tea, as Well as Green and Black (*Camellia sinensis*) Teas," *Mutation Research* 558, no. 1–2 (2004): 145–154. DOI: 10.1016/j.mrgentox.2003.12.003. https://www.sciencedirect.com/science/article/abs/pii/S1383571803003516.

59. L. Cai et al., "Purification, Preliminary Characterization and Hepatoprotective Effects of Polysaccharides from Dandelion Root," *Molecules* 22, no. 9 (2017): 1409. DOI: 10.3390/molecules22091409. https://www.mdpi.com/1420-3049/22/9/1409/htm.

60. B. A. Clare, R. S. Conroy, and K. Spelman, "The Diuretic Effect in Human Subjects of an Extract of *Taraxacum officinale* Folium over a Single Day," *Journal of Alternative and Complementary Medicine* 15, no. 8 (2009): 929–934. DOI: 10.1089/acm.2008.0152. https://www.ncbi.nlm.nih.gov/pmc/articles/PMC3155102/.

61. T. K. H. Chang, "Activation of Pregnane X Receptor (PXR) and Constitutive Androstane Receptor (CAR) by Herbal Medicines," *AAPS Journal* 11, no. 3 (2009): 590–601. DOI: 10.1208/s12248-009-9135-y. https://www.ncbi.nlm.nih.gov/pmc/articles/PMC2758128/.

62. J. Kiani and S. Z. Imam, "Medicinal Importance of Grapefruit Juice and Its Interaction with Various Drugs," *Nutrition Journal* 6, no. 33 (2007). DOI: 10.1186/1475-2891-6-33. https://www.ncbi.nlm.nih.gov/pmc/articles/PMC2147024/

63. B. H. Hellum, Z. Hu, and O. G. Nilsen, "Trade Herbal Products and Induction of CYP2C19 and CYP2E1 in Cultured Human Hepatocytes," *Basic & Clinical Pharmacology & Toxicology* 105, no. 1 (2009): 58–63. DOI: 10.1111/j.1742-7843.2009.00412.x. https://www.ncbi.nlm.nih.gov/pubmed/19371257.

64. M. K. Rasmussen, G. Zamaratskaia, and B. Ekstrand, "In Vivo Effect of Dried Chicory Root (*Cichorium intybus* L.) on Xenobiotica Metabolising Cytochrome P450 Enzymes in Porcine Liver," *Toxicology Letters* 200, no. 1–2 (2011): 88–91. DOI: 10.1016/j.toxlet.2010.10.018. https://www.ncbi.nlm.nih.gov/pubmed/21056093.

65. A. Ahmad et al., "A Review on Therapeutic Potential of *Nigella sativa*: A Miracle Herb," *Asian Pacific Journal of Tropical Biomedicine* 3, no. 5 (2013): 337–352. DOI: 10.1016/S2221-1691(13) 60075-1. https://www.ncbi.nlm.nih.gov/pmc/articles/PMC3642442/.

66. S. Hasani-Ranjbar, Z. Jouyandeh, and M. Abdollahi, "A Systematic Review of Anti-Obesity Medicinal Plants - An Update," *Journal of Diabetes & Metabolic Disorders* 12, no. 1 (2013): 28. DOI: 10.1186/2251-6581-12-28. https://www.ncbi.nlm.nih.gov/pubmed/23777875.

67. M. M. AbuKhader, "Thymoquinone in the Clinical Treatment of Cancer: Fact or Fiction?" *Pharmacognosy Review* 2013; 7, no. 14 (2013): 117–10. DOI: 10.4103/0973-7847.120509. https://www.ncbi.nlm.nih.gov/pmc/articles/PMC3841989/.

68. M. S. Touillaud et al., "Dietary Lignan Intake and Postmenopausal Breast Cancer Risk by Estrogen and Progesterone Receptor Status," *Journal of the National Cancer Institute* 99, no. 6 (2007): 475–486. DOI: 10.1093/jnci/djk096. https://www.ncbi.nlm.nih.gov/pmc/articles /PMC2292813/.

69. M. Ogata et al., "Supplemental Psyllium Fibre Regulates the Intestinal Barrier and Inflammation in Normal and Colitic Mice," *British Journal of Nutrition* 118, no. 9 (2017): 661–672. DOI: 10.1017/S0007114517002586. https://www.ncbi.nlm.nih.gov/pubmed/29185927.

Nourish Your Organs of Filtration: The Liver, Kidneys, and GI Tract

1. A. O. Docea et al., "Six Months Exposure to a Real Life Mixture of 13 Chemicals' Below Individual NOAELs Induced Non Monotonic Sex-Dependent Biochemical and Redox Status Changes in Rats," *Food and Chemical Toxicology* 115 (2018): 470–481. DOI: 10.1016 /j.fct.2018.03.052. https://www.sciencedirect.com/science/article/pii/S0278691518302011?via %3Dihub.

2. W. J. Chang et al., "The Relationship of Liver Function Tests to Mixed Exposure to Lead and Organic Solvents," *Annals of Occupational and Environmental Medicine* 25, no. 1 (2013): 5. DOI: 10.1186/2052-4374-25-5. https://www.ncbi.nlm.nih.gov/pmc/articles/PMC3886255/.

3. G. Malaguarnera et al., "Toxic Hepatitis in Occupational Exposure to Solvents," *World Journal of Gastroenterology* 18, no. 22 (2012): 2756–2766. DOI: 10.3748/wjg.v18.i22.2756. https://www.ncbi.nlm.nih.gov/pmc/articles/PMC3374978/.

4. Environmental Working Group, "State of American Drinking Water," https://www.ewg.org /tapwater/state-of-american-drinking-water.php#.WYDfkoqQwUE.

5. Environmental Protection Agency, "Consumer Confidence Reports," https://ofmpub.epa.gov /apex/safewater/f?p=136:102.

6. N. Tripathi, "The Disadvantages of Ion Exchange," *Sciencing*, April 25, 2017, https://sciencing .com/disadvantages-ion-exchange-8092882.html.

7. S. Dai, "Springbone, a Restaurant Dedicated to Bone Broth, Opens Friday in Greenwich Village," Eater New York, May 12, 2016, https://ny.eater.com/2016/5/12/11665206/springbone-bone-broth.

8. P. Diez, "Bone Broth Alchemist Marco Canora Opens West Village Brodo Dispensary," Eater New York, November 9, 2016, https://ny.eater.com/2016/11/9/13567014/brodo-west-village-opens.

9. S. Hall, "Bone Broth Is the New Coffee: Our Fave Paleo Staple Hits L.A.," The Chalkboard, April 21, 2015 http://thechalkboardmag.com/our-fave-paleo-staple-hits-l-a-bone-broth-is-the-new-coffee.

10. B. Holmes, "Chicken Soup for the Aging Star's Soul," ESPN, January 15, 2015 http://www.espn.com/nba/story/_/id/12168515/bone-broth-soup-helping-los-angeles-lakers-kobe-bryant.

Supplements for Keto Fasting

1. A. Fischer et al., "Coenzyme Q Regulates the Expression of Essential Genes of the Pathogen- and Xenobiotic-Associated Defense Pathway in *C. elegans*," *Journal of Clinical Biochemistry and Nutrition* 57, no. 3 (2015): 171–177. DOI: 10.3164/jcbn.15-46. https://www.ncbi.nlm.nih.gov/pmc/articles/PMC4639588/.

2. B. A. Daisley et al., "Microbiota-Mediated Modulation of Organophosphate Insecticide Toxicity by Species-Dependent Interactions with Lactobacilli in a *Drosophila melanogaster* Insect Model," *Applied and Environmental Microbiology* 84, no. 9 (2018). DOI: 10.1128/AEM.02820-17. https://www.ncbi.nlm.nih.gov/pubmed/29475860.

3. B. V. Deepthi et al., "*Lactobacillus plantarum* MYS6 Ameliorates Fumonisin B1-Induced Hepatorenal Damage in Broilers," *Frontiers in Microbiology* 8 (2017): 2317. DOI: 10.3389/fmicb.2017.02317. https://www.ncbi.nlm.nih.gov/pubmed/29213265.

4. S. Johnson, "The multifaceted and widespread pathology of magnesium deficiency," *Medical Hypotheses* 56, no. 2 (2001): 163–70. DOI: 10.1054/mehy.2000.1133. https://www.ncbi.nlm.nih.gov/pubmed/11425281

5. National Institutes of Health, "Magnesium: Fact Sheet for Health Professionals," https://ods.od.nih.gov/factsheets/Magnesium-HealthProfessional/.

6. National Center for Complementary and Integrative Health, "Milk Thistle," https://nccih.nih.gov/health/milkthistle/ataglance.htm.

7. D. S. Jaya, J. Augustine, and V. P. Menon, "Protective Role of N-acetylcysteine Against Alcohol and Paracetamol Induced Toxicity," *Indian Journal of Clinical Biochemistry* 9, no. 2 (1994): 64–71. DOI: 10.1007/BF02869573. https://link.springer.com/article/10.1007%2FBF02869573#page-1.

8. H. Sprince, "Protection against Acetaldehyde Toxicity in the Rat by L-Cysteine, Thiamin and L-2-Methylthiazolidine-4-Carboxylic Acid," *Agents and Actions* 4, no. 2 (1974): 125–130. DOI: 10.1007/BF01966822. https://link.springer.com/article/10.1007%2FBF01966822.

9. B. Olsson, "Pharmacokinetics and Bioavailability of Reduced and Oxidized N-Acetylcysteine," *European Journal of Clinical Pharmacology* 34, no. 1 (1988): 77–82. DOI: 10.1007/BF01061422. https://www.ncbi.nlm.nih.gov/pubmed/3360052.

10. L. Borgström, B. Kågedal, and O. Paulsen, "Pharmacokinetics of N-Acetylcysteine in Man," *European Journal of Clinical Pharmacology* 31, no. 2 (1986): 217-22. DOI: 10.10.07 /BF00606662. https://www.ncbi.nlm.nih.gov/pubmed/3803419.

11. M. M. Houck and J. A. Siegel, *Fundamentals of Forensic Science (Third Edition)* (San Diego: Academic Press, 2015), 155–179. DOI: 10.1016/B978-0-12-800037-3.00007-8. https://www.sciencedirect.com/science/article/pii/B9780128000373000078.

12. "MSM and Allergies," https://www.nutriteam.com/msm-allergies.

13. L. S. Kim et al., "Efficacy of Methylsulfonylmethane (MSM) in Osteoarthritis Pain of the Knee: A Pilot Clinical Trial," *Osteoarthritis and Cartilage* 14, no. 3 (2006): 286–94. DOI: 10.1016/j.joca .2005.10.003. https://www.ncbi.nlm.nih.gov/pubmed/16309928.

14. M. Butawan, R. L. Benjamin, and R. J. Bloomer, "Methylsulfonylmethane: Applications and Safety of a Novel Dietary Supplement," *Nutrients* 9, no. 3 (2017): 290. DOI: 10.3390 /nu9030290.

15. K. M. Dalessandri et al., "Pilot Study: Effect of 3,3'-Diindolylmethane Supplements on Urinary Hormone Metabolites in Postmenopausal Women with a History of Early-Stage Breast Cancer," *Nutrition and Cancer* 50, no. 2 (2004): 161–7. DOI: 10.1207/s15327914nc5002_5. https://www.ncbi.nlm.nih.gov/pubmed/15623462.

16. W. W. Zhang, Z. Feng, and S. A. Narod, "Multiple Therapeutic and Preventive Effects of 3,3'-Diindolylmethane on Cancers Including Prostate Cancer and High Grade Prostatic Intraepithelial Neoplasia," *Journal of Biomedical Research* 28, no. 5 (2014): 339–348. DOI: 10.7555/JBR.28.20140008. https://www.ncbi.nlm.nih.gov/pubmed/25332705.

17. H. L. Bradlow, "Review: Indole-3-Carbinol as a Chemoprotective Agent in Breast and Prostate Cancer," *In Vivo* (Athens, Greece) 22, no. 4 (2008): 441–5. https://www.ncbi.nlm.nih.gov /pubmed/18712169.

18. "British Scientists Have Developed Broccoli Pill to Help in Arthritis Fight," *Daily Express*, April 27, 2015. https://www.express.co.uk/life-style/health/573089/Broccoli-pill-help-arthritis-fight.

19. M. E. Sears, "Chelation: Harnessing and Enhancing Heavy Metal Detoxification—A Review," *Scientific World Journal* 2013: 219840. DOI: 10.1155/2013/219840. https://www.ncbi.nlm.nih .gov/pmc/articles/PMC3654245/.

20. J. Mikler et al., "Successful Treatment of Extreme Acute Lead Intoxication," *Toxicology and Industrial Health* 25, no. 2 (2009): 137–40. DOI: 10.1177/0748233709104759. https://www .ncbi.nlm.nih.gov/pubmed/19458136.

21. M. D. Aldridge, "Acute Iron Poisoning: What Every Pediatric Intensive Care Unit Nurse Should Know," *Dimensions of Critical Care Nursing* 26, no. 2 (2007): 43–8. https://www.ncbi.nlm.nih .gov/pubmed/17312404.

22. B. T. Ly, S. R. Williams, and R. F. Clark, "Mercuric Oxide Poisoning Treated with Whole-Bowel Irrigation and Chelation Therapy," *Annals of Emergency Medicine* 39, no. 3 (2002): 312–5. https://www.ncbi.nlm.nih.gov/pubmed/11867987.

23. M. N. V. R. Kumar, "A Review of Chitin and Chitosan Applications," *Reactive & Functional Polymers* 46, no. 1 (2000): 1–27. DOI: 10.1016/S1381-5148(00)00038-9. https://www .sciencedirect.com/science/article/abs/pii/S1381514800000389?via%3Dihub.

24. E. Guibal, "Interactions of Metal Ions with Chitosan-Based Sorbents: A Review," *Separation and Purification Technology* 38, no. 1 (2004): 43–7. DOI: 10.1016/j.seppur.2003.10.004. https://www.sciencedirect.com/science/article/pii/S1383586603002648.

25. A. J. Varmaa, S. V. Deshpandea, and J. F. Kennedy, "Metal Complexation by Chitosan and Its Derivatives: A Review," *Carbohydrate Polymers* 55, no. 1 (2004): 77–93. DOI: 10.1016/j.carbpol.2003.08.005. https://www.sciencedirect.com/science/article/pii/S0144861703002297.

26. L. Zhang, Y. Zeng, and Z. Cheng, "Removal of Heavy Metal Ions Using Chitosan and Modified Chitosan: A Review," *Journal of Molecular Liquids* 214 (2016): 175–191. DOI: 10.1016/j.molliq.2015.12.013. https://www.sciencedirect.com/science/article/pii/S0167732215308801.

27. J. Wang and C. Chen, "Chitosan-based biosorbents: Modification and application for biosorption of heavy metals and radionuclides," *Bioresource Technology* 160 (2014): 129–141. DOI: 10.1016/j.biortech.2013.12.110. https://www.sciencedirect.com/science/article/pii/S0960852413019500.

28. T. Fang et al., "Modified Citrus Pectin Inhibited Bladder Tumor Growth Through Downregulation of Galectin-3," Acta *Pharmacologica Sinica* 2018. DOI: 10.1038/s41401-018-0004-z. https://www.nature.com/articles/s41401-018-0004-z.

29. Z. Y. Zhao et al., "The Role of Modified Citrus Pectin as an Effective Chelator of Lead in Children Hos pitalized with Toxic Lead Levels," *Alternative Therapies in Health and Medicine* 14, no. 4 (2008): 34–8. https://www.ncbi.nlm.nih.gov/pubmed/18616067

30. I. Eliaz, E. Weil, and B. Wilk, "Integrative Medicine and the Role of Modified Citrus Pectin/Alginates in Heavy Metal Chelation and Detoxification—Five Case Reports," *Forschende Komplementärmedizin* 14, no. 6 (2007): 358-64. DOI: 10.1159/0000109829. https://www.ncbi.nlm.nih.gov/pubmed/18219211.

31. Oregon State University, "Chlorophyll and Chlorophyllin," https://lpi.oregonstate.edu/mic/dietary-factors/phytochemicals/chlorophyll-chlorophyllin.

32. J. Berry, "What Are the Benefits of Chlorophyll?" Medical News Today July 4, 2018, https://www.medicalnewstoday.com/articles/322361.php.

33. C. Xu et al., "Light-Harvesting Chlorophyll Pigments Enable Mammalian Mitochondria to Capture Photonic Energy and Produce ATP," *Journal of Cell Science* 127 (2014): 388–99. DOI: 10.1242/jcs.134262. https://www.ncbi.nlm.nih.gov/pubmed/24198392.

Supporting Your Keto Fast with Sauna Therapy

1. S. J. Genuis et al., "Human Elimination of Phthalate Compounds: Blood, Urine, and Sweat (BUS) Study," *Scientific World Journal* 2012: 615068. DOI: 10.1100/2012/615068. https://www.ncbi.nlm.nih.gov/pmc/articles/PMC3504417/.

2 S. J. Genuis et al., "Human Excretion of Bisphenol A: Blood, Urine, and Sweat (BUS) Study," *Journal of Environmental and Public Health* 2012: 185731. DOI: 10.1155/2012/185731. https://www.hindawi.com/journals/jeph/2012/185731/.

3. CBS News, "Toxic Metal Cadmium Found in Chain Stores' Jewelry for Adults," October 11, 2018, https://www.cbsnews.com/news/toxic-metal-cadmium-found-in-chain-stores-jewelry-for-adults/.

4. M. E. Sears, K. J. Kerr, and R. I. Bray, "Arsenic, Cadmium, Lead, and Mercury in Sweat: A Systematic Review," *Journal of Environmental and Public Health* 2012:184745. DOI: 10.1155/2012/184745. https://www.hindawi.com/journals/jeph/2012/184745/.

5. S. J. Genuis et al., "Blood, Urine, and Sweat (BUS) Study: Monitoring and Elimination of Bioaccumulated Toxic Elements," *Archives of Environmental Contamination and Toxicology* 61, no. 2 (2011): 344–357. DOI: 10.1007/s00244-010-9611-5. https://link.springer.com /article/10.1007%2Fs00244-010-9611-5

6. A. Kenttämies and K. Karkola, "Death in Sauna," *Journal of Forensic Sciences* 53, no. 3 (2008): 724–729. DOI: 10.1111/j.1556-4029.2008.00703.x. https://www.ncbi.nlm.nih.gov/pubmed /18471223.

INDEX

ACKNOWLEDGMENTS

My deepest appreciation for the two primary editors who helped create this book. Kate Hanley is a brilliant, kind, and talented writer who skillfully helped craft my recommendations into text.

Janet Selvig was the other primary editor. Janet is my sister, and I love her dearly. She started my medical practice with me in 1985, and was my first employee. She continues to work as the chief editor of our website. I can always count on her to give me honest and highly insightful edits. I don't know what I would do without her.

— Dr. Joseph Mercola

ABOUT THE AUTHORS

Dr. Joseph Mercola

Dr. Joseph Mercola is a physician and *New York Times* best-selling author. He was voted the Ultimate Wellness Game Changer by the Huffington Post and has been featured in several national media outlets, including *Time* magazine, the *Los Angeles Times*, CNN, Fox News, ABC News, *TODAY*, and *The Dr. Oz Show*. His mission is to transform the traditional medical paradigm in the United States into one in which the root cause of disease is treated, rather than the symptoms. In addition, he aims to expose corporate and government fraud and mass media hype that often sends people down an unhealthy path. Website: mercola.com

Pete Evans

Pete Evans, host of the WGBH series *Moveable Feast with Fine Cooking*, is an award-winning Australian chef, restaurateur, cookbook author, and TV personality. Pete's food career began when he and his brother Dave opened their first restaurant, The Pantry, in Melbourne in 1993. It quickly became a much-loved and critically acclaimed local spot. Since then, Pete has opened six award-winning restaurants and written seven best-selling cookbooks, including the Australian barbecue bible *My Grill*. He has hosted television shows in Australia for the past decade, and in 2012, his series *My Kitchen Rules* pulled an audience of more than 3.5 million, making it one of the most-watched shows of the year in Australia. Website: peteevans.com

HAY HOUSE TITLES OF RELATED INTEREST

YOU CAN HEAL YOUR LIFE, *the movie,* starring Louise Hay & Friends
(available as a 1-DVD program, an expanded 2-DVD set,
and an online streaming video)
Learn more at www.hayhouse.com/louise-movie

THE SHIFT, *the movie,* starring Dr. Wayne W. Dyer
(available as a 1-DVD program, an expanded 2-DVD set,
and an online streaming video)
Learn more at www.hayhouse.com/the-shift-movie

——

THE ALLERGY SOLUTION: *Unlock the Surprising Hidden Truth about
Why You Are Sick and How to Get Well,* by Leo Galland, M.D.

COMPLETE KETO: *A Guide to Transforming Your Body
and Your Mind for Life,* by Drew Manning

FEEDING YOU LIES: *How to Unravel the Food Industry's
Playbook and Reclaim Your Health,* by Vani Hari

YOUNG AND SLIM FOR LIFE: *10 Essential Steps to Achieve Total Vitality
and Kick-Start Weight Loss That Lasts,* by Dr. Frank Lipman

All of the above are available at your local bookstore,
or may be ordered by contacting Hay House (see next page).

——

We hope you enjoyed this Hay House book. If you'd like to receive our online catalog featuring additional information on Hay House books and products, or if you'd like to find out more about the Hay Foundation, please contact:

Hay House, Inc., P.O. Box 5100, Carlsbad, CA 92018-5100
(760) 431-7695 or (800) 654-5126
(760) 431-6948 (fax) or (800) 650-5115 (fax)
www.hayhouse.com® • www.hayfoundation.org

———

Published in Australia by:
Hay House Australia Pty. Ltd., 18/36 Ralph St., Alexandria NSW 2015
Phone: 612-9669-4299 • *Fax:* 612-9669-4144 • www.hayhouse.com.au

Published in the United Kingdom by:
Hay House UK, Ltd., Astley House, 33 Notting Hill Gate, London W11 3JQ
Phone: 44-20-3675-2450 • *Fax:* 44-20-3675-2451 • www.hayhouse.co.uk

Published in India by: Hay House Publishers India,
Muskaan Complex, Plot No. 3, B-2, Vasant Kunj, New Delhi 110 070
Phone: 91-11-4176-1620 • *Fax:* 91-11-4176-1630 • www.hayhouse.co.in

———

Access New Knowledge.
Anytime. Anywhere.

Learn and evolve at your own pace
with the world's leading experts.

www.hayhouseU.com

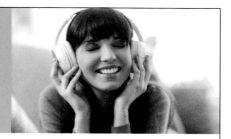

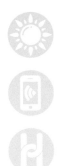

Hay House Podcasts
Bring Fresh, Free Inspiration Each Week!

Hay House proudly offers a selection of life-changing audio content via our most popular podcasts!

Hay House Meditations Podcast

Features your favorite Hay House authors guiding you through meditations designed to help you relax and rejuvenate. Take their words into your soul and cruise through the week!

Dr. Wayne W. Dyer Podcast

Discover the timeless wisdom of Dr. Wayne W. Dyer, world-renowned spiritual teacher and affectionately known as "the father of motivation". Each week brings some of the best selections from the 10-year span of Dr. Dyer's talk show on HayHouseRadio.com.

Hay House World Summit Podcast

Over 1 million people from 217 countries and territories participate in the massive online event known as the Hay House World Summit. This podcast offers weekly mini-lessons from World Summits past as a taste of what you can hear during the annual event, which occurs each May.

Hay House Radio Podcast

Listen to some of the best moments from HayHouseRadio.com, featuring expert authors such as Dr. Christiane Northrup, Anthony William, Caroline Myss, James Van Praagh, and Doreen Virtue discussing topics such as health, self-healing, motivation, spirituality, positive psychology, and personal development.

Hay House Live Podcast

Enjoy a selection of insightful and inspiring lectures from Hay House Live, an exciting event series that features Hay House authors and leading experts in the fields of alternative health, nutrition, intuitive medicine, success, and more! Feel the electricity of our authors engaging with a live audience, and get motivated to live your best life possible!

Find Hay House podcasts on iTunes, or visit www.HayHouse.com/podcasts for more info.

HAY HOUSE
Online Video Courses

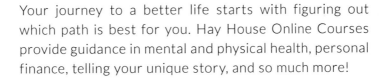

Your journey to a better life starts with figuring out which path is best for you. Hay House Online Courses provide guidance in mental and physical health, personal finance, telling your unique story, and so much more!

LEARN HOW TO:

- choose your words and actions wisely so you can tap into life's magic

- clear the energy in yourself and your environments for improved clarity, peace, and joy

- forgive, visualize, and trust in order to create a life of authenticity and abundance

- break free from the grip of narcissists and other energy vampires in your life

- sculpt your platform and your message so you get noticed by a publisher

- use the creative power of the quantum realm to create health and well-being

To find the guide for your journey, visit www.HayHouseU.com.

HAY HOUSE
online learning